SKIN BIOPSY - DIAGNOSIS AND TREATMENT

Edited by **Suran L. Fernando**

Skin Biopsy - Diagnosis and Treatment
http://dx.doi.org/10.5772/46018
Edited by Suran L. Fernando

Contributors

Maria Azul Montani, Gisela Vaglio Giors, Khitam Al-Refu, Suran Fernando, Olga L. Bohn, Sergio Sanchez-Sosa, Julie Teruya-Feldstein

Published by InTech

Janeza Trdine 9, 51000 Rijeka, Croatia

Publishing Process Manager Ana Pantar
Technical Editor InTech DTP team
Cover InTech Design team

Additional hard copies can be obtained from orders@intechopen.com

Skin Biopsy - Diagnosis and Treatment, Edited by Suran L. Fernando
p. cm.
ISBN 978-953-51-1173-3

For EU product safety concerns:
IN TECH d.o.o., Prolaz Marije Krucifikse Kozulić 3, 51000 Rijeka, Croatia,
info@intechopen.com or visit our website at intechopen.com.

Meet the editor

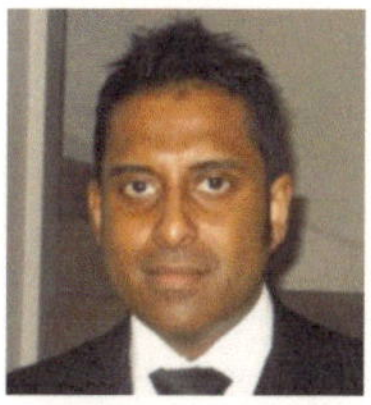

Dr. Suran Fernando is a Clinical Immunologist and Immunopathologist. He is a Clinical Associate Professor of Medicine at the Sydney Medical School, University of Sydney, Australia, the Inaugural Head of the Department of Clinical Immunology and Allergy at Royal North Shore Hospital, Sydney, the Medical Director of HIV Services in the Northern Sydney Local Health District, and the Manager of the ImmunoRheumatology Laboratory of the Sydney Division of Pathology North. Dr. Fernando graduated from the University of New South Wales, Sydney in 1994 with honours and obtained fellowships of the Royal Australasian College of Physicians and Royal College of Pathologists of Australasia, respectively, in 2001. He completed his doctoral thesis in 2005 in the Mycobacterial Laboratory at the Centenary Institute, Sydney, under the supervision of Prof. Warwick Britton, studying the p2x7 purinergic receptor and mycobacterial infections in humans. Since his appointment to Royal North Shore Hospital in 2008, he has strengthened the Discipline of Immunology though the provision of a thriving tertiary referral inpatient and outpatient service, the establishment of specialty clinics such as drug testing and neuroimmunology clinics, the introduction of in vitro drug allergy tests, and training and research programs for specialty registrars and scientists. He is on several advisory and policy forming committees including the New South Wales HIV and Sexually Transmitted Infections Strategic Planning Committee, The Australasian Society Clinical Immunology and Allergy Anaphylaxis Working Party, The Australasian Society Clinical Immunology Stinging Insect Working Party, The Australian and New Zealand Anaesthetic Allergy Group, and The International Mentoring Program of the Australasian Society of HIV Medicine. Dr. Fernando's range of research interests includes drug allergy, autoimmune bullous diseases, neuroimmunology, and the relationship between infection and immunity. He has over 100 publications in the form of peer-reviewed articles, invited reviews, books, book chapters, and published abstracts.

Contents

Preface

It is with pleasure that I present this book, Skin Biopsy – Diagnosis and Treatment.

Skin Biopsy– Diagnosis and Treatment is a collection of six chapters. The initial chapter on Site Selection by Maria Azul Montani and Gisela Vaglio Giors illuminates the importance of site selection as means of optimizing the utility of skin biopsy in the diagnosis of various dermatological diseases and in many instances it is a therapeutic intervention and is useful in monitoring the response to therapy. This is the first article to explore such a topic is depth.

The next five chapters encompass the application and role of skin biopsy to the overall diagnosis of certain conditions. An accurate diagnosis allows for an up to date discussion on the treatment of these complex conditions as the pathogenesis and the histologic findings are evolving and the therapeutic options are concomitantly emerging. Khitam Al-refu describes in detail the technique of scalp biopsy and its role in the diagnosis of non-scarring and scarring alopecia. Olga Bohn et al. reveal the clinical manifestations, histopathology, immunoprofile, electron microscopic and molecular features of Langerhans cell neoplasms of the skin, a field, which is rapidly evolving with the advances in technological applications used in the skin tumors. I review and update the reader on the epidemiology, nosology, diagnostic criteria, pathogenesis, and treatment of Stevens-Johnson syndrome/toxic epidermal necrolysis, Drug Reaction Eosinophilia and Systemic Symptoms/Drug Induced Hypersensitivity Syndrome, and acute generalized exanthematous pustulosis that comprise severe cutaneous adverse reactions. With Jamma Li, I provide the latest review on the pathogenesis, histology, and treatment options for pemphigus vulgaris and foliaceus. Mark Schifter writes the final chapter by lending his expertise to the classification, pathogenesis, histology and treatment for oral lichen planus.

I am grateful to the other authors for their excellent contributions to this book. I am incredibly indebted to the InTech team for all their efforts in making this publication possible and widely accessible to the interested public. In particular, I would like to thank Ana Pantar from InTech for her tireless dedication, organisation, patience and faultless assistance in the preparation of this book.

Suran L. Fernando
Royal North Shore Hospital and Sydney Medical School,
Sydney University
Sydney, Australia

Chapter 1

Site Selection

Maria Azul Montani and Gisela Vaglio Giors

Additional information is available at the end of the chapter

http://dx.doi.org/10.5772/55638

1. Introduction

Skin biopsy is a fundamental method to correct diagnosis in lots of skin diseases. To make a "good use" of it, it is necessary to know at what time, to whom it can be done, how many biopsies, and principally in which sites can be applied.

Once choosing the biopsy site, it must be taken into account several factors that depend on the patient and the type of lesion concerned. Also, it should be considered the elementary type of lesion, the depth of it, and the indemnity of the skin as well as other factors.

Within the type of lesions, there are certain diseases that have special features when the physician decide make biopsy such as pigmented lesions and alopecia.

The skin biospies are extremely useful not only for diagnosis, but also for monitoring, therapy evaluation and sometimes they are the treatment itself for certain skin diseases.

In recent times there have been studies that are used in skin biopsies for the diagnosis and /or follow up of non-dermatological diseases, such as neuropathies and intravascular lymphoma B cells. In these diseases there are not typical or no typical cutaneous lesions. Therefore, it is in these cases when we ask where it would be the most suitable site to take the biopsy.

2. Body

The selection of the site of biopsy depends on two factors which can be classified as: patient-dependent and dependent on the skin lesion.

Among the factors are patient-dependent which we describe as sex, age, skin type and reception of treatments for the condition we are evaluating. Sex and age differences implicate structural skin and variations in thickness or degree of photoaging, treatments received, such as the use of corticosteroids, may also generate changes. All the above factors are interrelated, since age is inversely proportional to the thickness, broadly photoaging is also associated with age and affects the thickness of the skin, as if the patient is receiving treatment corticoid by parenteral, oral or local cause, a decrease in thickness and increase cutaneous capillary fragility, which could modify the histopathological appearance of skin biopsy.

Besides skin region where the lesion is located is another factor to consider when choosing the biopsy site, as this last point can vary the amount of annexes found, as hair follicles, sebaceous and sweat glands, the presence of previous scars or the presence of inflammatory or reactive changes unrelated to the underlying disease, such as stasis dermatitis in the legs may become evident.

Whenever possible, the operator should take samples from several representative sites on the trunk or proximal extremities, given that skin on the distal lower extremities nearly always shows a degree of inflammatory infiltrate and changes related to superimposed stasis dermatitis; moreover, surgical wounds in distal areas will heal more slowly. [1]

Another more trivial aspect but not less important in some patients, especially in women, is whether the lesion is in a region more or less visible, is not the same to make a skin biopsy in the face or neck than in the abdomen, if it is located on the face or neck it will be convenient to perform the procedure in a way that the possible scar will be the smallest. One shave biopsy is possibly the most likely form of modality used for this area. [2]

Then there are the factors dependent of the skin lesion, first of all, it is essential to select a representative area of the lesion devoid of artefact, it is different taking a biopsy from a tumor than from an ulcer.

With regard to this, when choosing the biopsy site it should be taken into account the type of elementary lesion involved and its evolution time (it depends on the type of lesion, its evolution and the place where the skin biopsy is taken.[3]

For example, in the case of ulcers, biopsy must be performed in the edge of it trying to cover healthy skin, and bottom edge of the ulcer; and in the case of annular lesions, such as granuloma annulare, dermatomycosis, erythema chronicum migrans, erythema annulare centrifugum, cutaneous lupus erythematosus, porokeratosis and others, tissue must be sampled from the active border, in the case of a lump or lesion that is felt more than seen, indicating that it is located in the dermis and / or subcutaneous tissue, it should be done in the deepest part. As shown, each elementary lesion involves certain characteristics that modify the selection of the site from which the biopsy will be taken. **See Table 1.**

A factor to consider at the moment of doing the skin biopsy, is the **level of the lesion in the skin**. In case of lesions located in epidermis and papillary dermis such as melanocytic nevus, age spots, seborrheic keratosis, fibroepithelial polyps, common wart, superficial basal cell carcinoma, melanoma in situ, mycosis fungoides, actinic keratosis, Paget disease (mammary and extramammary), contact dermatitis (allergic and irritant), atopic dermatitis, seborrheic dermatitis, plaque psoriasis, scabies, lichen planus, Gibert pityriasis rosacea and vesiculobullous dermatosis. The skin biopsy should include epidermis and a bit of dermis.

http://dx.doi.org/10.5772/55638

Disease	Time	Site selection
Alopecia areata	Active	Border
Telogen efluvium	Active	Most hairless
Alopecia scarring	Active	Erythematous, follicular plugs, inflamed follicule
Alopecia paraneoplastica	Suspicious papule	Center
Atopic or contact dermatitis	Acute	Erythematous skin vesicle
	chronic	Lichenified areas
Exanthema	Active	Lesion
Erythema annulare centrifugum	Well-developed lesion	Active border
Erythema multiforme	Targetoid lesion	One from dusky center; one from the erythematous border
Erythema nodosum and all panniculitides	Active lesion, first week	Center
Fascitis	Active	Center
Granuloma annulare	Active	Raised border
Larva migrans	Migrating erythema	Normal skin 2mm above the tip of erythematous line
Lichen planus	Any time	Violaceous papule
Lupus erythematosus discoid	Active lesion	Erythematous scaly plaque with follicular plugs
Lupus tumidus	Active lesion	Anywhere
Lupus erythematosus, subacute cutaneous	Active lesion	Anywhere
Lupus erythematous systemic	Active	Anywhere
Lupus profundus	Depressed center and adjacent area	Center
Mycosis fungoides	1- Patche stage, untreated lesion	1- Center
	2- Plaque stage, non-ulcerated	2- Most infiltrated area
	3- Tumor stage, non-ulcerated	3- Indurated area
Morphea	1- Early	1- Lilac ring
	2- Late	2- Center
Necrobiosis lipoidica	Anytime	Ivory atrophic center, avoid bony area
Nephrogenic fibrosing dermopathy	Sclerotic plaques	Indurated area or sclerotic plaque and normal-appearing skin
1- Parapsoriasis large plaque	1- and 2- any stages	1- Untreated lesion
2- Parapsoriasis small plaque		2- Center
Pityriasis lichenoides chronica	2-3 weeks old	Papulosquamous papule
PLEVA	2-3 weeks old	Necrotic papule
Psoriasis guttate	Late stage	Lesional
Psoriasis plaque	Scaly	Anywhere

Disease	Time	Site selection
Psoriasis pustular	Early pustule	Anywhere
Pyoderma gangrenosum and ulcerative disease	Small, early non-ulcerated lesion	Entire lesion
Scabies	Non-infected	Proximal edge of burrow
Scleromyxedema	Sclerotic skin	Beaded papules
Tinea corporis	Untreated, if possible	Erythematous raised border
Tinea pedis	Untreated, if possible	Vesicular or scaly border
Urticaria and urticarial vasculitis	Active 3 days	Lesional

Table 1. Add caption

If it involves papillary and reticular dermis the technique must include these layers, these lesions are melanocytic nevus, glomus tumor, neurofibroma, hemangioma, sebaceous nevi, follicular cysts, basal cell carcinoma (solid, sclerodermiform), melanoma, squamous cell carcinoma, photoallergic dermatitis, phototoxic dermatitis, polymorphic light eruption, scleroderma, morphea, scabietic nodules, leukocytoclastic vasculitis, cutaneous lupus erythematosus, urticaria, granuloma annulare.

If they involve reticular dermis and subcutaneous tissue the biopsy has to be deeper, these lesions are blue nevus, lipoma, dermatofibroma, epidermoid or trichilemmal cysts, melanoma, cuteaneous lymphoma, dermatofibrosarcoma protuberans, metastasis (melanoma, breast cancer), panniculitis, sarcoidosis, rheumatoid nodules, nodular vasculitis, polyarteritis nodosa, thrombophlebitis, granuloma annulare. [4]

In skin diseases that manifest with multiple lesions, once the physician performs complete physical examination of the patient along with a complete history he/she will choose the lesion to perform the biopsy. He/she will observe the most recent lesions, the most representative ones, in which no treatment was done, medically indicated or not, and if it is an evidence of more than one type of elementary lesion, he/she will decide to make as number of biopsies as types of lesions are present. If several specimens are obtained from different lesions or appearance of different ages, these should be placed in different and appropriately labelled containers. [3]

In addition, if an **infectious process** is suspected, then part of the tissue should always be submitted for microbiology studies to identify bacteria, mycobacteria, fungi and viruses. [3]

As stated, skin biopsies must contain adequate specimen to include the three basic components of the skin, but this depends on several aspects, a factor taken into account for this to be possible, is the indemnity of lesional and perilesional skin, whether it is friable or soft it is more likely that at the time of the procedure is difficult to show the three layers of the skin in the histopathological examination. If it is hard or fibrous, it is more difficult to accomplish but it is easier to show the various layers of the skin. The ideal lesion to be biopsied is the harmless and / or without signs of infection, it is sometimes difficult to be like this way because in the case of patients with pruritic lesions they can be infected by scratching. For these reasons, it is advisable that before performing skin biopsy, the lesion should be evaluated and if necessary,

http://dx.doi.org/10.5772/55638

prescribe antibiotics or local anti-inflammatories and after these take effect, do the same. It is also common for patients that self-medicate or those who use different free sold medications that modify the appearance of the lesion.

We note that an **untreated lesion** should be selected for biopsy, or in addition, one should discontinue therapy for one week (if possible) before taking the biopsy. [3]

When someone performs a skin biopsy with diagnostic purposes, for therapeutic monitoring or therapeutic evaluation it should not be always done on skin lesions, it can also be done on normal skin, this happens in cases of experimental studies in which healthy skin should be compared with affected skin. Also, biopsy of healthy skin close to skin lesions when you suspected vasculitis or bullous disease such as bullous pemphigoid, epidermolysis bullosa acquisita, pemphigoid gestationis, cicatricial pemphigoid, dermatitis herpetiformis, pemphigus or some kind of non bullous diseases that may present blisters as lupus erythematosus or lichen planus, for direct immunofluorescence seeking deposits of antibody as IgG, IgA, IgM, C3, fibrin, or complexes antibody- antigen. [3][5][6] This assay should be performed in lesions that have less than 24 hours of evolution, since otherwise it is difficult to observe the presence of immunocomplexes and there are only reactive changes. [6]

Certain pathologies involve a careful choosing of the biopsy site, such as pigmented lesions and alopecia.

Excisional biopsy should be performed in pigmented lesions, but in some cases it can´t be done, the most representative area would be selected. [6] The skin biopsy is the fundamental tool of the dermatologist to evaluate the nature of a pigmented lesion. Clinical examination and dermatoscopy are currently the two widely utilized modalities for examination of pigmented lesions. [2]

In a randomized controlled trial, dermatoscopy added to routine physical examination was also shown to decrease the number of biopsies without decreasing the number of melanomas that were detected. [7] There are 3 major techniques for the biopsy of a pigmented lesion: shave biopsy, punch/incisional biopsy, and excisional biopsy. [8]

The decision to biopsy a pigmented lesion rests principally on the clinician's experience; dermoscopy is useful too. When deciding whether to biopsy or not, Bolognia has said that in case of pigmented lessions the first step is visualizing the gross configuration of the tumor as well as a cross-section of the skin that contains the tumor cells. Thus, an important part of the physical examination is palpation of the suspicious lesion. Due to the fact that a melanoma with invasion feels thicker than a melanoma in situ, palpation can aid in the selection of the biopsy method. [8][9]

In case of multiple pigmented lesions the most unusual appearing lesion is the one that must be taken the biopsy. Guidelines of the British Association of Dermatologists indicate that excisional biopsy of clinically suspicious lesions is almost always preferable to any other technique. And they note that each clinical scenario relies on decision making that takes many factors into account.[10]

The American Academy of Dermatology has recently issued a position statement on the management of melanoma, recommending that a narrow excisional biopsy with 1 mm to 3 mm margins is required to clear the subclinical component of most atypical melanocytic lesions and it is therefore preferable in almost all scenarios. [11] When performing a shave biopsy of a pigmented lesion, the best is to remove the diameter of the lesion completely, otherwise the biopsy is considered a partial biopsy and the true nature of the lesion cannot be ascertained with accuracy by the examining pathologist. If a lesion is large and biopsy of the entire area would leave a significant scar, it is better to biopsy the darkest or most unsual part of the lesion. [8] Another remarkable aspect of the shave method is to provide good cosmetic outcome, as we described before.

Incisional biopsies have been recommended in other circumstances, including extensive or large pigmented lesions with unclear margins, extensive facial lentigo maligna, pigmented lesions in acral areas, and pigmented lesions in mucosal areas. [12] Somach et al study found a diagnostic discordance between incisional and excisional biopsy of about 40% in lesions evaluated. This finding indicates that the portion of the lesion most worrisome to a clinician may not correspond to the most histologicaly aggressive portion of a melanocytiv lesion. [13] The disadvantage of the incisional biopsy technique is overcalling the lesion as a melanoma when it is not, [8] or missing the diagnosis of a melanoma.

The gold standard for melanoma diagnosis is excisional biopsy, and it should be performed on any lesion that is highly suspicious for melanoma. One way to select the site or the size of the excisional biopsy is using a Wood's lamp to detect subclinical pigmentation. The orientation is along the relaxed skin tension lines and the draining lymphatics from the site. This orientation theoretically allows a more accurate sentinel lymph node biopsy if it is later needed. On the extremities it is preferable to orient such excisions vertically rather than horizontally to preserve better the lymphatic architecture. [8]

When the decision to biopsy melanonychia is made, there are 3 main methods to do: a 3-mm punch biopsy, a shave biopsy, or a fusiform excision to the periostium. Although the most widely accepted one is a longitudinal full-thickness excisional procedure, given that shave biopsies fail to evaluate the thickness of the lesion. [14] Before obtaining a biopsy, the nail plate is viewed end-on with dermoscopy, because lesions that are present in the dorsal nail plate reflect a melanocytic origin at the proximal nail matrix, whereas lesions presented in the ventral nail plate correspond to origin at the distal nail matrix [2]

Various choices for biopsy are available depending on the presence of Hutchinson's sign, width and location of the nail band, and the origin within the matrix of the nail band. Regardless of the biopsy type, pain management and control of bleeding are paramount. [2]

When melanoma is highly suspected in a pigmented band, nail biopsy should include as much of the longitudinal band, including periosteum, as possible. Ideally, the proximal nailfold and nail plate should both be reflected to allow visualization of the origin of the melanonychia. For lesions smaller than 3 mm, a telescoping punch biopsy technique can be used. [2]

When the pigmented lesion is in the lips the site selection depends on the location of it. On the cutaneous lip, a shave biopsy is acceptable if the lesion does not cross the vermilion border. [8]

http://dx.doi.org/10.5772/55638

On the mucosal lip, a punch biopsy is preferred. [8] If the pigmented lesion crosses the vermilion border, a punch biopsy should be performed with orientation vertically. The border of the lip should be marked with a gentian violet marking pen so that when the suture is placed to close the defect, the border can be aligned precisely. [8]

Scalp skin biopsies are frequently performed for evaluation of the classification and patogénesis of **alopecias**. Two 4-mm punch biopsy specimens, both submitted in buffered formalin, are required: one for vertical (longitudinal) sections, and the other for transverse (cross) sections. If only one specimen is available, it is bisected vertically, one side (cut side down) for vertical sectioning and the other side sectioned at 1mm below the skin surface, both pieces are embedded with sides cut down for serial sections. [3] There are limitations in interpreting scalp skin biopsies in both vertical and cross sections: biopsy site selection is critical; the histopathologic features of several end-stage alopecias cannot be distinguished and a 4 to 6mm biopsy sample may not be representative of the entire scalp area. [3] In suspected cicatricial alopecia a sample should be sent to histopathology and another one to perform immunofluorescence. [6]. In cicatricial alopecias, mainly cutaneous lupus erythematosus and lichen planus, the biopsy must be performed in an active margin, trying to choose the edge of the activity or scar areas and (ideally no more than one third of the surface area should correspond to scar). [6]

Another factor to consider in choosing the biopsy site is the goal of it, because it could be for diagnosis, monitoring or treatment. In case it is diagnostic, the site selection and depth varies according to the type of elementary lesion concerned, but in most cases the center of the lesion is the chosen place.

When the biopsy is for diagnosis, it always should, regardless of the method that is done, try to cover the three layers of skin: epidermis, dermis and hypodermis. This last layer is essential especially in nodular lesions, more palpable than visible.

Rajaratnam et al revised 100 skin biopsies and in 78% of the cases, histology with the aid of clinical information was able to provide an accurate diagnosis correlating to the working diagnosis. [15]

The skin biopsy has been reported to be of varying usefulness in making a diagnosis. [15][16]

As stated earlier the biopsy site will depend on the type of elementary lession, but in general, incisional biopsy is preferred and will be at the center of the tumor and inflammatory lesions, in the annular rim of annular lesions and shall include center and border in ulcers areas. In the case of pigmented lesions excisional biopsy is preferred.

When a biopsy is performed to follow a disease is suggested to do it in the same place as the biopsy was made to diagnose, not exactly at the same, but as close as you can, because if done in the exact place, only scar tissue will be evident in histopathological examination. Skin biopsy for this purpose is not necessary to do as a routine procedure, but it is indicated when the underlying disease is malignant and treatment of it was just local, it is carried out to assess whether it was successful or not. It can also be used as a tool for non-responsive dermatoses. Another plausible case for the biopsy is when the first diagnosis was basal cell carcinoma or squamous cell carcinoma and in the time of definitive treatment initial lesion can not be found, a second biopsy was performed at the site of the first or adjacent to it, to make the right treatment.

In most instances, the purpose of the biopsy is diagnostic or monitoring, but often ends up being therapeutic,in spite of the fact that it hasn´t been the main objective. That is, for example, when the lesions are small, that is to say entering in a punch of 6 mm or less. It has also been described in cases of basal cell carcinoma or keratoacanthoma in which after diagnostic biopsy at the time of definitive treatment, is not even the primary lesion biopsied. On these cases a second biopsy must be performed to do the correct treatment. In cases where no lesion was found, the biopsy ended up being therapeutic without being this its first target. [17]

Laboratories in Europe and the USA have increasingly included skin biopsy in the diagnosis assessment or follow-up of patients with **Peripherals neuropathy.** [18] When a skin biopsy is done with this purpose, it can be done at any site of the body. A 3 milimeters diameter punch is commonly used with no need for sutures. For diagnostic purpose, one skin biopsy is commonly done at a distal site on the leg (10 cm above lateral malleolus) and a further biopsy taken at a proximal site on the thigh (20 cm below the iliac spine); thus a proximal site and a distal site can be compared if a length-dependent process is suspected. Skin biopsy can also be done in other regions of the body (eg. Face, trunk, or fingers). [18]

Skin biopsy is a safe, minimally invasive, painless and cheap tool to provide diagnostic information on small nerve fibers, which are invisible to routine neurophysiological tests. Sommer et al in his experience with more than 1000 biopsy samples, he discovered that there were not side-effects or complaints. Healing in those cases was usually complete within one week, and barely visible scar usually remains. [18] Biopsy can be performed in hairy skin to investigate unmyelinated and thinly myelinated fibers and in glabrous skin to examine large myelinated fibers. [19]

One further advantage of skin biopsy over conventional nerve biopsy is that it allows somatic nerve fibers to be distinguished from autonomic nerve fibers. Morphological changes, axonal degeneration and abnormal regeneration occur in cutaneous nerves very early in the course of peripheral neuropathies, making skin biopsy a promising tool to investigate the progression of neuropathy and the effect of neuroprotective treatments in clinical practice and trials.[19]

The neuropathies in which the skin biopsy is useful are diabetic neuropathy [18], demyelinating neuropathies like Charcot-Marie-Tooth disease. [20][21], neuropathy associated with systemic diseases including sarcoidosis, systemic lupus erythematosus, Sjögren's syndrome, celiac disease, and Friedreich's ataxia and Fabry's disease. [22][23][24][25]. Infectious and inflammatory neuropathies like leprosy, HIV-associated sensory neuropathy, Churg Strauss syndrome. [26][27].

In diabetic neuropathy, skin biopsy is the most sensitive measureof a charge in the severity of neuropathy. [18] Monitoring method is an useful to track the progression of neuropathy in trials of neuroprotective treatments. In case of using skin biopsy to monitor progression or evaluate the effect of neuroprotective treatments; it should be repeated close to the site of a previous biopsy, within the territory of the same sensory nerve [19]Another use of blind skin biopsy is in the diagnosis of **intravascular B-cell lymphoma**. This lymphoma is a rare one and its diagnoses turns really difficult so blind skin biopsy is an option for diagnosis.

Cutaneous manifestations of intravascular large B-cell lymphoma are nonspecific and appear as edema, peau d'orange, nodules, patches, plaques, and/or telangiectasias and can mimic common lesions such as thrombophlebitis, livedo, or vasculitides. [28] These skin lesions are the result of malignant lymphocytes distributed heterogeneously throughout the papillary and reticular dermal vascular plexuses. [28][29].

Le et al describes the use of blind skin biopsy in this type of lymphoma and despite the absence of cutaneous findings, skin biopsy specimens were obtained. There are limited data on how often blind skin biopsy specimens yield positive results in intravascular large B-cell lymphoma, and there are no guidelines on which sites to choose or how many biopsies to perform. [30] One way to select the site of biopsy is reviewing the frequency depending on location, a recent review reported: thigh (41%), leg (35%), trunk (31%), arm (15%), and buttock (7,5%).[28] Based on this review, biopsy specimens from the case of Le et al were taken from the front of the thighs bilaterally, with 3 of the 4 revealing intravascular large B-cell lymphoma. [30] They have done more than one biopsy because of the small size of the biopsy specimen itself. The skin biopsy is a valuable and minimally invasive diagnostic tool that should be considered for patients with a high index of suspicion for intravascular large B-cell lymphoma, even in the abscense of cutaneous findings. [30]

Sjoberg et al described another use of skin biopsy, it can be useful to remove sea urchin spines.

A biopsy punch with a diameter of 2 mm was used to cut out each spine including a small piece of surrounding dermal tissue to support the fragile remmants of calcium carbonate. [31]

Sjoberg et al exposed that a dermal biopsy punch, commonly found in most medical offices, is a simple and handy tool to solve this problem and thereby reducing the morbidity of the patient [31]

In these cases, site selection is exactly where the urchin spine is located.

3. Conclusion

In our search for information on the most suitable biopsy sites and stage of disease for optimal pathologic diagnosis, we did not find any article devoted entirely to this subject. Only sketchy information was available. Skin biopsy is an accessible tool, easy to perform, inexpensive, relatively safe and allows us to access the histopathological examination of the skin in all its depth, all layers, and microbiological studies or immunofluorescence or immunohistochemistry can be made from it. This diagnostic method is for the dermatologist what the blood test is for the clinicians. Notably, its basic use, the most important and widely disseminated is in the diagnosis of various skin diseases, but it can also be used in monitoring and therapeutic evaluation of these diseases. For its easy carrying and accessibility, its application has been described in the diagnosis of non-dermatological diseases such as peripheral neuropathy, innovative application, which is deployed on multiple research studies, and offers a less invasive and easy –to-perform tool for the diagnosis of this pathology.

Author details

Maria Azul Montani and Gisela Vaglio Giors

Department of Dermatology, Hospital Italiano de Buenos Aires, Argentina

References

[1] Pinkus, H. Skin biopsy: a field of interaction between clinician and pathologist. Cutis. (1977). , 20-609.

[2] Tran, K, Wright, N, et al. biopsy of the pigmented lesion-When and how. Journal American Academy of Dermatology (2008). , 59(5), 852-71.

[3] Sina, B, Kao, G, et al. Skin biopsy for inflammatory and common neoplastic skin diseases: optimum time, best location and preferred techniques. A critical review. Journal of Cutaneous Pathology. (2009). , 36-505.

[4] Llamas-velasco, M, & Paredes, E. Basic Concepts in skin biopsy. Part I. Actas dermosifiliográficas. (2012). , 103(1), 12-20.

[5] Fitzpatrick

[6] Llamas-velasco, M, & Paredes, B. La biopsia cutánea: bases fundamentales. Parte II. Actas Dermo-Sifiliográficas. (2012). , 103(2), 100-10.

[7] Carli, P, De Giorgi, V, et al. Addition of dermoscopy to conventional naked-eye examination in melanoma screening: a randomized study. Journal American Academy of Dermatology (2004). , 50-683.

[8] Silverstein, D, & Mariwalla, K. Biopsy of pigmented lesions. Dermatological Clinical (2012). , 30-435.

[9] Bolognia, J. Biopsy techniques for pigmented lesions. Dermatological Surgery (2000). , 26(1), 89-90.

[10] Marsden, R, Newton-bishop, J, et al. Revised UK guidelines for the management of cutaneous melanoma 2010. Journal Plastic Reconstruction Aesthesia Surgery (2010). , 63(9), 1401-19.

[11] Bichakjian, C, Halpern, A, et al. Guidelines of care for the management of primary cutaneous melanoma. Journal American Academy of Dermatology (2011). , 65(5), 1032-47.

[12] Pflugfelder, A, Weide, B, et al. Incisional biopsy and melanoma prognosis: facts and controversies. Clinical Dermatology (2010). , 28(3), 316-8.

[13] Somech, S, Taira, J, et al. Pigmented lesions in actinically damaged skin. Histopathologic comparison of biopsy and excisional specimens. Archives of Dermatology (1996). , 132(11), 1297-302.

[14] Connor, O, & Dzwierzynski, E. W. Longitudinal melonychia, clinical evaluation and biopsy technique. Journal Hand Surgery American (2011). , 36(11), 1852-4.

[15] Rajaratnam, R, Smith, A, et al. The value of skin biopsy in inflammatory dermatoses. American Journal of Dermatopathology. (2009). , 31(4), 350-53.

[16] Nicolis, G, & Helwig, E. Exfoliative dermatitis: a clinicopathological study of 135 patients. Archives Dermatology. (1973). , 79-788.

[17] Marini M

[18] Sommer, C, & Lauria, G. Skin biopsy in the management of peripheral neuropathy. Lancet Neurology (2007). , 6-632.

[19] Lauria, G, & Devigili, G. Skin biopsy as a diagnostic tool in peripheral neuropathy. Nature Clinical Practice Neurology. (2007). , 3(10), 546-57.

[20] Bai, J, Ghandour, K, et al. Skin biopsies in myelin-related neuropathies: bringing molecular pathology to the bedside. Brain (2005). , 128-1168.

[21] Sabet, A, Ghandour, K, et al. Skin biopsies demonstrate MPZ splicing abnormalities in Charcot-Marie- Tooth neuropathy 1B. Neurology (2006). , 67-1141.

[22] Nolano, M, Provitera, V, et al. Small fibers involvement in Friedreich's ataxia. Annals of Neurology (2001). , 50-17.

[23] Hoitsma, E, Marziniak, M, et al. Small fibre neuropathy in sarcoidosis. Lancet (2002). , 359-2085.

[24] Goransson, L, Herigstad, A, et al. Peripheral neuropathy in primary Sjögren's syndrome: a population-based study. Archives of Dermatology (2006). , 63-1612.

[25] Scott, L, Griffin, J, et al. Quantitative analysis of epidermal innervatrion in Fabry disease. Neurology (1999). , 52-1249.

[26] Herrmann, D, Mcdermott, M, et al. Epidermal nerve fiber density, axonal swellings and QST as predictors of HIV distal sensory neuropathy. Muscle Nerve (2004). , 29-420.

[27] Herrmann, D, et al. Is skin biopsy a predictor of transition to symptomatic HIV neuropathy? A longitudinal study. Neurology (2006). , 66-857.

[28] Roglin, J, & Böer, A. Skin manifestations of intravascular lymphoma mimic inflammatory diseases of the skin. British Journal of Dermatology (2007). , 157-16.

[29] Ponzoni, M, & Ferreri, A. Intravascular lymphoma: a neoplasm of "homeless" lymphocytes? Hematologic Oncology. (2006). , 24-105.

[30] Le, E, Gerstenblith, M, et al. The use of blind skin biopsy in the diagnosis of intravascular B-cell lymphoma. Journal American Academy of Dermatology. (2008). , 59(1), 148-51.

[31] Sjoberg, T, & De Weerd, L. The usefulness of a skin biopsy punch to remove sea urchin spines. Journal Compilation of Royal Australasian Colege of Surgeons. (2010).

Chapter 2

Scalp Biopsy and Diagnosis of Common Hair Loss Problems

Khitam Al-refu

Additional information is available at the end of the chapter

http://dx.doi.org/10.5772/55025

1. Introduction

Patients presenting with hair loss (alopecia) is a very common problem and is often a cause of great concern for cosmetic and psychological reasons and this has several causes; as it may be an important sign of systemic disease.

2. Causes of alopecia

Alopecia can be either scarring or non-scarring. Non-scarring alopecias tend to have preserved follicular ostia, with no clinically visible inflammation in most presentations, although histologic inflammation may be present. The common types of non-scarring alopecias are androgenic alopecia, telogen effluvium, alopecia areata, trichotillomania and traction alopecia. Scarring alopecias, also known as cicatricial alopecia, refers to a collection of hair loss disorders that have loss of follicular ostia, or atrophy, with permanent and irreversible destruction of hair follicles and their replacement with scar tissue. The histologic confirmation is the best method to confirm the presence of a fibrosing/scarring process with loss of hair follicles.

Scarring alopecias can be classified as lymphocytic (discoid lupus erythematosus (DLE), lichen planopilaris (LPP), central centrifugal cicatricial alopecia, pseudopelade of Brocq), neutrophilic (folliculitis decalvans, dissecting folliculitis), and mixed (acne keloidalis) entities [1].

Many alopecia types are biphasic. For example, androgenetic alopecia eventually results in loss of ostia and thus may appear like a scarring alopecia.

To establish the cause of the hair loss, one requires a history to identify known triggers, scalp examination, biochemical investigations and in many cases histology to identify the earliest stages of some types of alopecias esp scarring alopecia.

3. Indications of scalp biopsy in diagnosis of hair loss

Scalp biopsies can be used to make or confirm a diagnosis of alopecia. Scalp biopsy is considered mandatory in all cases of scarring alopecia. The interpretation of the histopathological findings of primary scarring alopecias without known clinical history may be difficult and this is especially true if the biopsy specimen is inadequate.

In non-scarring type, it is not difficult to diagnose these disorders. However, scalp biopsy can be needed in few cases of:

- Lack of identifiable triggers.
- Severe hair loss (as in some cases of alopecia areata which does not present in a well defined bald area, but as severe hair loss (Fig 1).
- Acute hair loss.
- Telogen effluvium does not occur in an acute way after a known triggering factor.
- Some cases of female androgenetic alopecia pattern; the clinical presentation may be similar to other types of non-scarring alopecias.

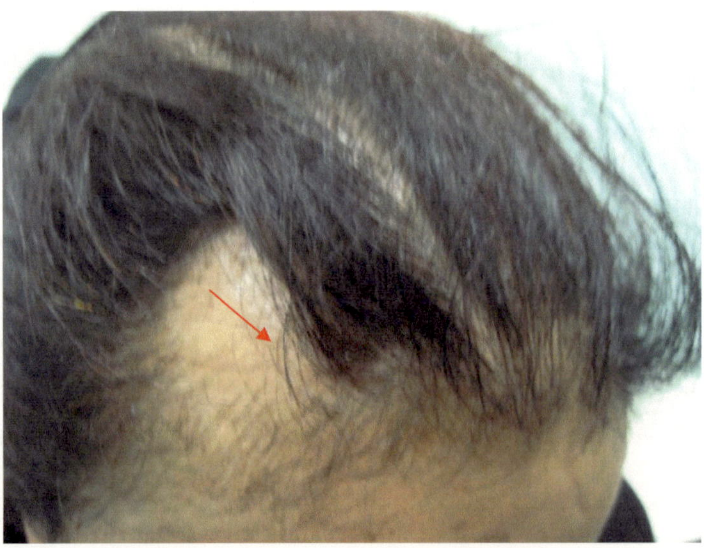

Figure 1. year old female patient presented with diffuse, acute severe hair loss and with localized patch of alopecia areata as it demonstrated by red arrow.

4. Technique of scalp biopsy

It is a crucial to determine the appropriate site of a scalp biopsy to have a correct diagnosis of alopecia, and this approach is different in scarring and non-scarring types. For a scarring process, the biopsy should be taken from the active border of hair loss where some hairs still remain and are more likely to display diagnostic findings. For non-scarring alopecias, the preferred site of biopsy is generally the border of a lesion (positive exclamation marks in alopecia areata), or from the site of a positive pull test in the setting of a diffuse alopecia. In the setting of evaluating a possible androgenic alopecia, two biopsies, one from the involved scalp (often vertex) and one from the uninvolved scalp (often occiput; serves as a positive control) may be beneficial.

The current gold-standard for a scalp biopsy specimen is the use of a 4-mm punch and must include subcutaneous fat to ensure sampling of the entire follicular unit and any anagen follicles; the specimen may be sectioned vertically or transversely [2]. Although a combination of the two may be optimal, the pathologist is frequently only provided with a single specimen.

5. Vertical sections

Vertically-sectioned punch biopsy specimen is adequate for assessing alopecias associated with interface changes, lichenoid infiltrates, and subcutaneous pathology [3]. However, vertical sectioning will show only 10% of the follicles present in the specimen [4]because the hair follicles, which grow at an angle, cannot be visualized in their entirety in conventional vertical sections.

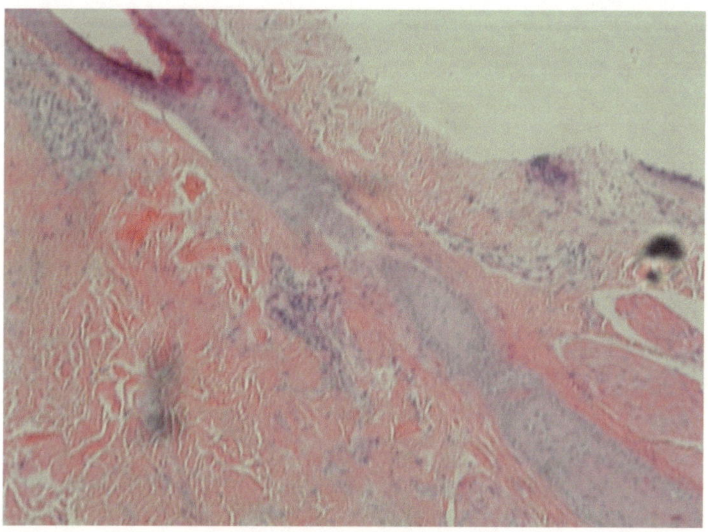

Figure 2. Vertical section of a scalp biopsy from a patient with DLE.

6. Horizontal sections

Horizontal sections are becoming the method of choice as they offer the advantage of evaluating large numbers of follicles simultaneously, determining hair density, location of inflammatory infiltrate and anagen to telogen ratio [5]. A transversely sectioned specimen will include all the hair follicles present in the biopsy, and in the same section. Although the clinical impression is very important in diagnosing alopecia, transversely sectioned biopsy specimens can greatly aid the diagnosis and management of patients with alopecia [6].

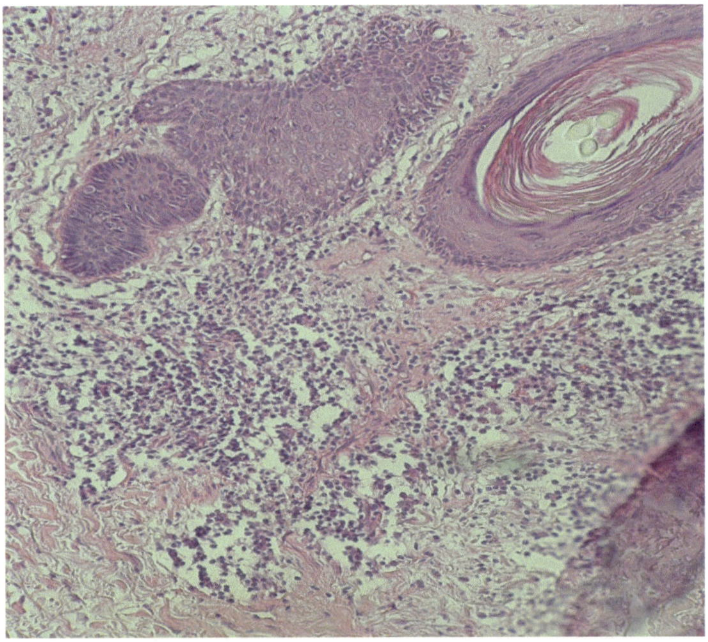

Figure 3. Transverse section from a scalp biopsy from a patient with DLE.

7. Hematoxylin and eosin staining of scalp biopsy

The histological findings in many forms of hair loss may be similar, and an accurate diagnosis of hair loss depends on distinguishing abnormal from normal follicular architecture. It is important to identify the normal hair follicle structure, the number, size and distribution of hair follicles within a biopsy specimen. Hematoxylin and eosin staining of the scalp biopsies is the usual satin in most of the cases of hair loss, but in some of the alopecias (such as DLE), immunofluorescence staining may be needed to add in diagnosis. In addition, the pathologist may use additional special stains to narrow a differential diagnosis or confirm an initial impression and one of these is immunohistochemistry which is dependent on the localization

http://dx.doi.org/10.5772/55025

of antigens in tissue sections by the use of labeled antibody as specific reagents through antigen-antibody interactions that are visualized by a marker such as peroxidase.

8. Histopathological findings in different types of hair loss

Specimens are categorized as scarring or nonscarring alopecia, and further diagnostic criteria discussed herein assist the pathologist in making specific diagnoses of nonscarring and scarring alopecias.

9. Scarring alopecia

Histologically, cicatricial alopecia is characterized by dermal scarring, along with absent or reduced hair follicles and reduced number of erector pili muscles. But taking skin biopsy from the active area will be more informative about the diagnosis.

This scarring alopecia may be secondary, and due to numerous etiologies (such as due to infectious causes (Fig 4), or primary, where the cause and pathogenesis are largely unknown, but the target is the hair follicle itself (such as DLE and LPP).

The discussion in following sections is about the primary type as the skin biopsy is more informative about the diagnosis.

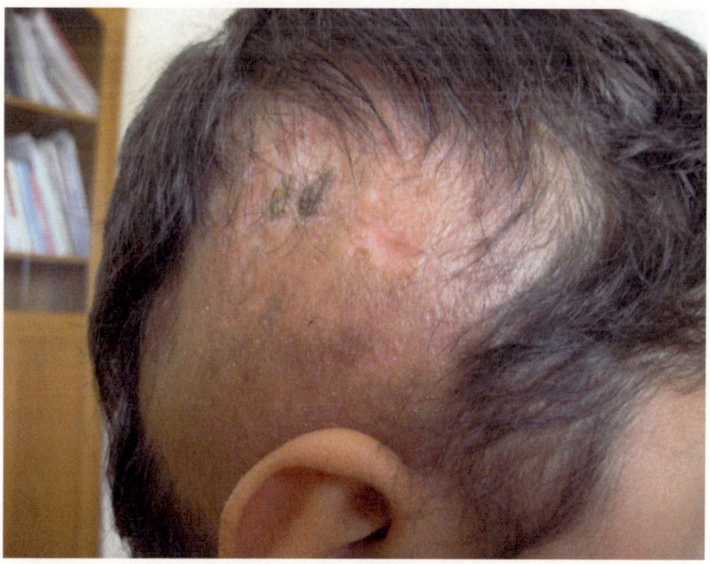

Figure 4. Scarring alopecia in a child secondary to tinea capitis.

10. Lupus erythematosus

Lupus erythematosus is an autoimmune disease that can affect one or more internal organs as well as the skin. This disease is a clinical spectrum ranging from mildly affected patients with only localized skin disease to those at risk of dying from systemic manifestations. The skin involvement is among the most frequent symptoms; and is characterized by its natural history of relapsing and chronicity. The scalp (Fig 5) is a common area of involvement, and permanent alopecia may result with the following morphological features; sclero-atrophy, erythema, follicular hyperkeratosis, plugging and telangiectasia. The irreversible, scarring alopecia differs from the reversible non scarring alopecia that is seen in patients with systemic lupus erythematosus.

Scarring alopecia in DLE may mimic other types of scarring alopecia seen in some dermatoses, the most common differential diagnosis of this is lichen planopilaris (LPP) and the differentiation between them is possible by early clinical and histological changes. Both LPP and DLE show perifollicular erythema and keratotic follicular papules, but the distinctive clinical features of DLE of the scalp are the presence of erythema, scaling, telangiectasia, and mottled hyperpigmentation within the areas of scarring alopecia and the presence of hyperkeratotic papules in the central part of the bald area in DLE, while in LPP it presents at the margin of the alopecia patch [7].

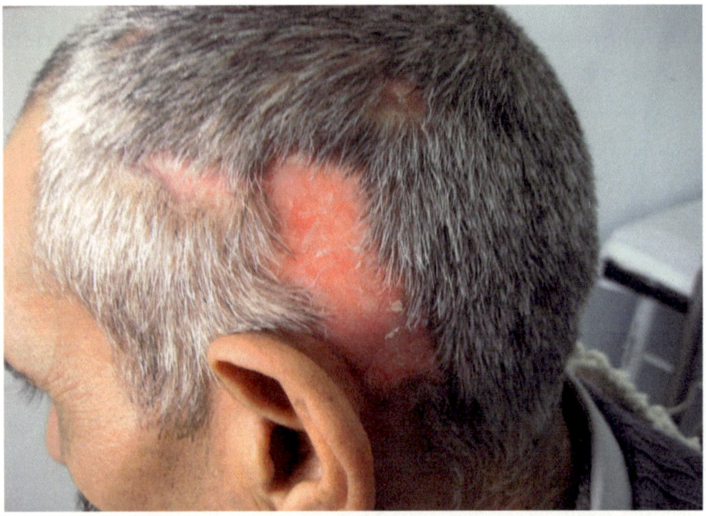

Figure 5. Discoid lupus erythematosus of the scalp. The typical scaling is evident.

DLE is a scarring disease and so early treatment is needed to control existing cutaneous lesions and limit scaring and to prevent the development of the disease. Patients with DLE lesions should have regular clinical evaluation accompanied by simple laboratory studies to evaluate the possible progression from the primary cutaneous disorder to the disorder accompanied by systemic involvement. Therapy begins with general measures such as the use of sun-protective measures, including sunscreens, protective clothing and medical therapy includes corticosteroids (topical or intralesional) and antimalarials.

Routine histologic examination of lesional skin from CLE patients is necessary, as the diagnosis of CLE generally requires clinicopathologic correlation and the distinction between different types of CLE based on histological findings without clinical correlation is difficult; all forms of CLE are similar histologically in broad terms. Histopathological features (Fig 6) include pilosebaceous atrophy, hyperkeratosis, parakeratosis, basement membrane thickening, subepidermal oedema and vasodilatation. A perivascular and peri-appendageal superficial and deep lymphoid cell infiltrate with plasma cells are other histolopathological findings.

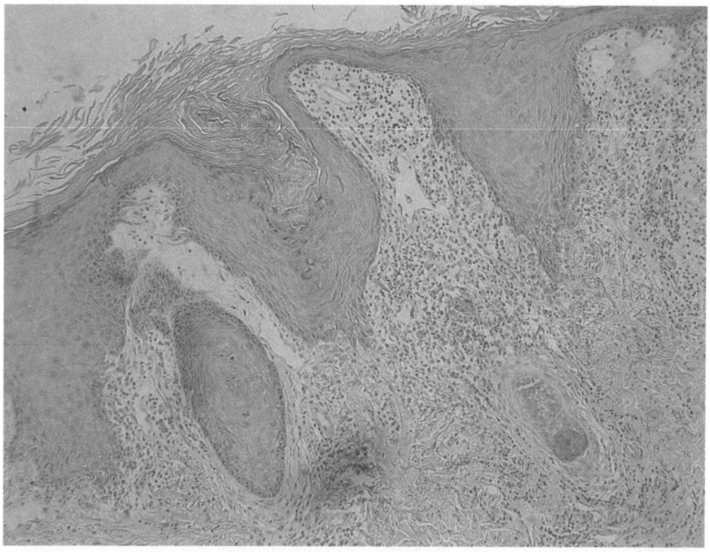

Figure 6. DLE pathology. Note the hyperkeratosis, basal cell degeneration and heavy inflammatory infiltrate.

Direct immunofluorescence (DIF) of lesional skin in CLE is an adjunctive test; it helps to confirm the diagnosis when the routine histological findings are equivocal. The test is positive only in some of lesional skin biopsies; so light microscopy should be carried out before DIF. For DIF, the optimal lesion of LE should be an established, erythematosus lesion, and of at least 6-8 weeks in duration. The most suggestive findings are the presence of multiple immunoreactants typically IgG and IgM, in a special pattern (bright in intensity, continuous, perifollicular, and granular) [8]. Sometimes complement components may be present including C3b and C1q. Scalp lesions have been reported to show the highest frequency of the DIF test (83 %), the immunoreactants deposits occur around hair follicles, an important feature not seen in other types of scarring alopecia.

Using immunohistochemistry [9], there were significant alterations in the basement membrane zone (BMZ) in patients with active DLE and this explain the previous histological findings of thickened BMZ in DLE. There was an increase in the expression of the anchoring fibril and collagen component antigens in the BMZ with gross thickening and protrusion into the dermis in active DLE lesions (Fig 7).

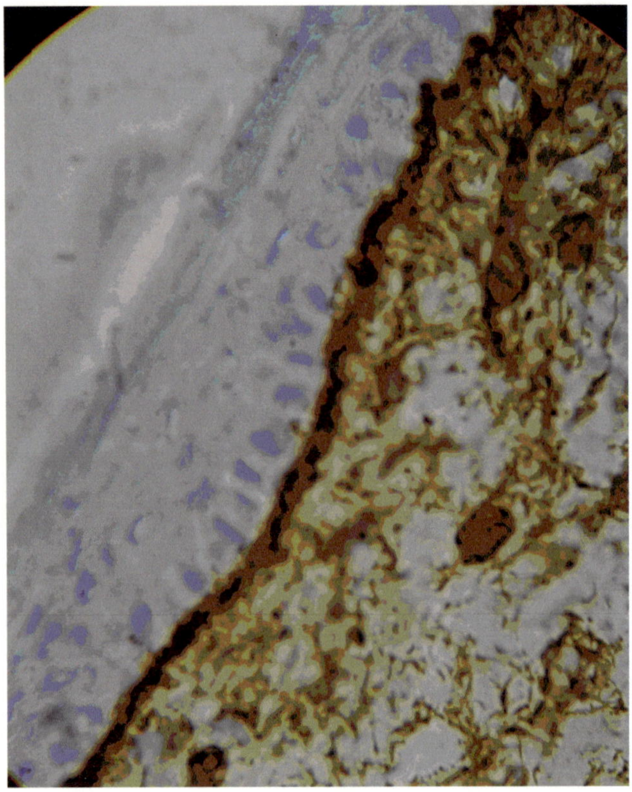

Figure 7. Anti-type IV collagen staining in DLE with an exaggerated expression as demonstrated by thickness of the basement membrane and protrusions.

11. Lichen Planopilaris (LPP)

LPP is a rare type of lichen planus which characteristically affects the scalp (Figure 8) with perifollicular erythema, keratotic follicular spines and with patchy or diffuse hair loss which may result in scarring alopecia as its end stage. Scalp lesions can be associated with characteristic flat topped violaceous papules of lichen planus (LP) on the limbs in 50 % of cases [10]. LPP of the scalp is a scarring disease and it is difficult to treat comparing to the glabrous LP and this has major psychological consequences for the affected patients. The therapeutic management often is quite challenging, as relapses are common after local or systemic treatments. The recommended treatments are ultrapotent topical or intralesional injections of corticosteroid. Some cases may need systemic treatment including oral corticotherapy and cyclosporine.

http://dx.doi.org/10.5772/55025

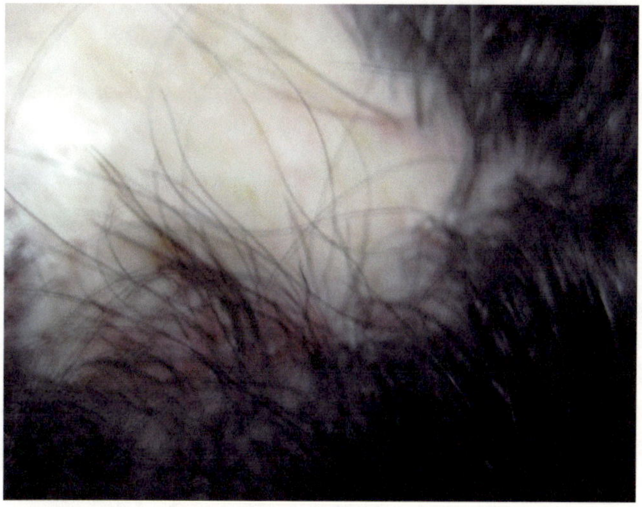

Figure 8. LPP of the scalp.

Histologically (Fig 9) has been reported to show two different patterns [11], each pattern characterized by the presence of specific histological features that reflects the specific stage of the progression of the disease. In the first pattern, hair follicles and the perifollicular dermis were mainly involved in the pathologic process, with no involvement of the interfollicular structures. In the second pattern, the pathologic changes extended to the interfollicular epidermis and the papillary dermis.

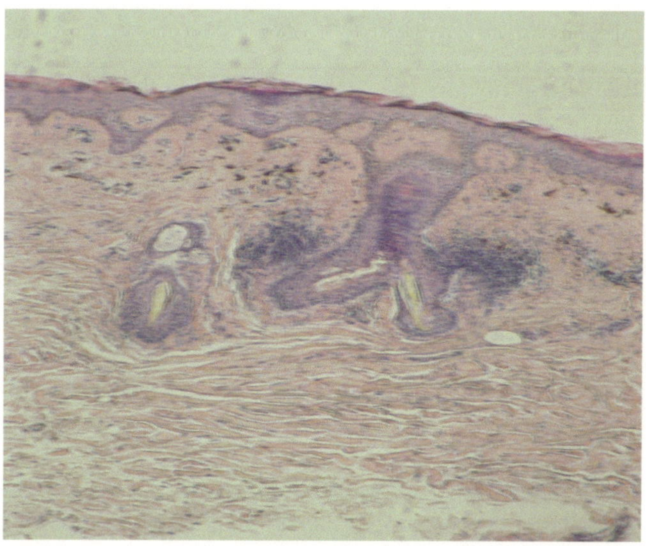

Figure 9. LPP pathology. The inflammation is mainly perifollicular with some involvement of the basal cell layers which also show basal cell degeneration.

Direct immunofluorescence highlights the presence of colloid bodies in the peri-infundibular area staining with IgM (less frequently with IgG, IgA and C3).

By immunohistochemistry staining [12], there is a significant alteration in the basement membrane structure in lesions of LPP which could differentiate it from active lesions of scalp DLE lesions.

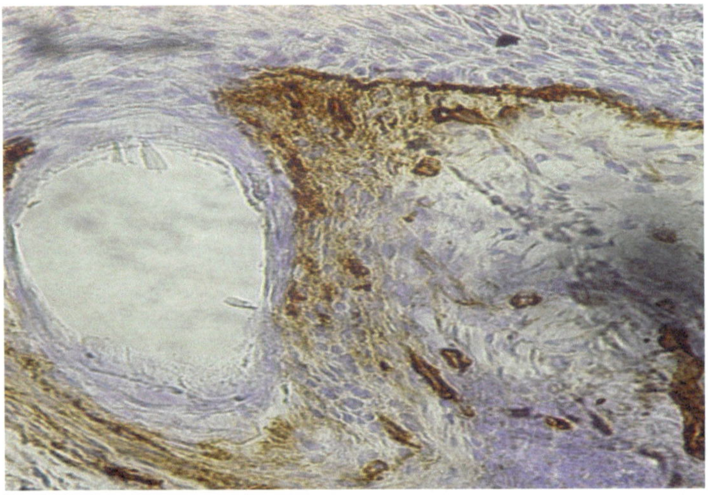

Figure 10. Anti-type IV collagen staining in LPP. Interrupted expression of type IV collagen in an affected hair follicle in an LPP lesion with projections into the underlying dermis, with the adjacent epidermis showing normal expression of the collagen

12. Non scarring alopecia

The diagnosis of this type of alopecia is usually based on a thorough history and a focused physical examination. In some patients, punch biopsy may be necessary if the cause of hair loss is unclear as has been described previously. The focus in the following discussion will be on alopecia areata and androgenetic alopecia (the skin biopsies will be needed in some of cases).

13. Alopecia Areata

Alopecia areata (Fig 11) is one form of non-scarring alopecia characterize by patchy hair loss of autoimmune origin. It usually presents as a single or multiple confluent patches of non-scarring alopecia. Spontaneous regression of the disease is common in this disease and the hair may grow back if the affected region is small. Topical treatment is effective including corticosteroids clobetasol or fluocinonide, corticosteroid injections, or cream, steroid injections,

http://dx.doi.org/10.5772/55025

topical minoxidil, irritants (anthralin or topical coal tar), and topical immunotherapy. Oral corticosteroids decrease the hair loss, but only for the period during which they are taken.

Diagnostic pathological findings (Fig 12) are more prominent in this type of alopecia which characterize by peribulbar lymphocytic inflammation which is usually considered to be an essential finding in establishing the diagnosis [13]. The lymphocytic

infiltrate is rich in helper T cells, which are considered to be evidence of an autoimmune process. Despite this, it may be absent in many scalp biopsy specimens. In the acute stage; a moderate to dense inflammatory cell infiltrate (mainly lymphocytes and langerhans cells) [14] develops around anagen hair and this leads finally to anagen arrest and inhibition which weakens the lowest portion of the

hair shaft. Using follicular counts [15] related to the stage of disease is a useful way to establish the histologic features of alopecia areata in scalp biopsy specimens taken from different types of alopecia areata; alopecia areata should be suspected when high percentages of telogen hairs are present, even in the absence of a peribulbar infiltrate [15].

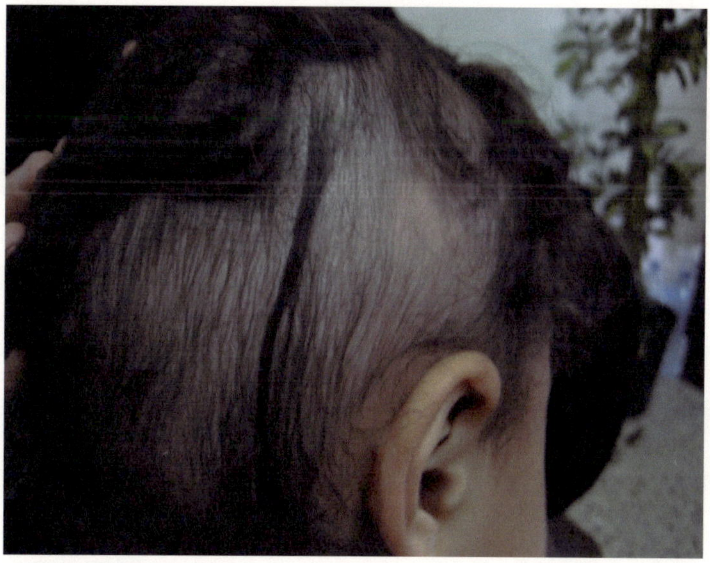

Figure 11. Alopecia areata in a child presented with diffuse hair loss.

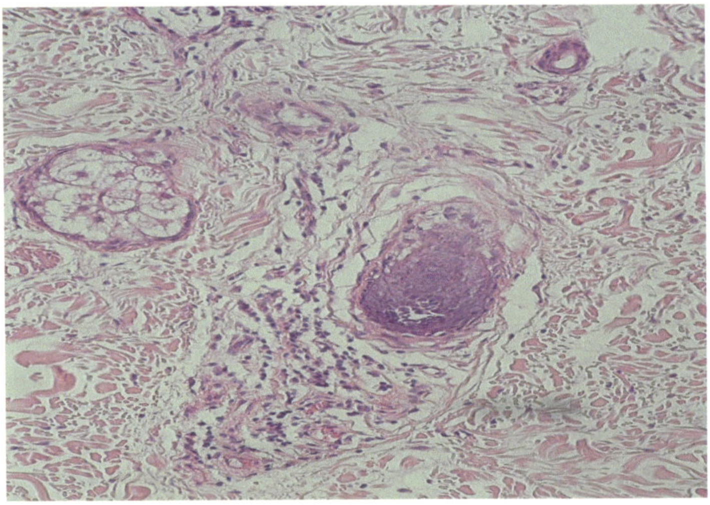

Figure 12. Skin biopsy from a patient with alopecia areata demonstrating perifollicular lymphocytic infiltrate.

14. Androgenetic alopecia

Androgenic alopecia is the most common type of hair loss. Clinically, it is a patterned alopecia, in that it is characterized by bitemporal recession and vertex balding in men, and in women (female pattern hair loss) by diffuse hair thinning of the crown with an intact frontal hairline. Histopathologically, the use of transverse sections is the most valuable method to reach a diagnosis [16], as all the hair follicles can be visualized.

The terminal (T) to vellus (v) ratio is T: V= less than 4:14. Normal scalp ratio is T: V= 7:1). A ratio of T: V= 3: 1 or less is considered to be diagnostic [16], [17].

Author details

Khitam Al-refu

Faculty of Medicine, Mu'tah University, Jordan

References

[1] Olsen EA, Bergfeld WF, Cotsarelis G et al. Summary of North American Hair Research Society (NAHRS)-sponsored Workshop on Cicatricial Alopecia, Duke Univer-

sity Medical Center, February 10 and 11, 2001. J. Am. Acad. Dermatol. 2003; 48; 103–110.

[2] Elston DM, Ferringer T, Dalton S, Fillman E, Tyler W. A comparison of vertical versus transverse sections in the evaluation of alopecia biopsy specimens. J Am Acad Dermatol. 2005 Aug;53(2):267-72.

[3] Frishberg DP, Sperling LC, Guthrie VM. Transverse scalp sections: a proposed method for laboratory processing. J. Am. Acad. Dermatol. 1996; 35; 220–222.

[4] Headington JT. Transverse microscopic anatomy of the human scalp. A basis for a morphometric approach to disorders of the hair follicle. Arch. Dermatol. 1984; 120; 449–456.

[5] Whiting D: The value of horizontal sections of scalp biopsies. J Cutan Aging Cosmetic Dermatol 1:165-173, 1990.

[6] Templeton SF, Santa Cruz DJ, Solomon AR. Alopecia: histologic diagnosis by transverse sections. Semin Diagn Pathol. 1996 Feb;13(1):2-18.

[7] Fabbri, P. Amato, L., Chiarin, C., Morretti, S. & Massi, D. (2004). Scarring alopecia in discoid lupus erythematosus: a clinical, histopathologic and immunopathologic study. *Lupus* 13(6), 455-462.

[8] Costner, M.I. & Sontheimer, R.D. (2003). Skin manifestations of rheumatologic multisystem diseases: Lupus erythematosus. *In*: Freedberg, I.M. *et al*, *Fitzpatrick's Dermatology in general medicine*. Sixth edn. 1677-1776.

[9] Al-refu k & Goodfield M. Immunohistochemistry of ultrastructural changes in scarring lupus erythematosus. Clin exp Dermatol. 2011. 36, 36-8.

[10] Mehregan, D., Van Hale, H. &Muller, S. (1992). Lichen planopilaris: clinical and pathologic study of forty-five patients. *J Am acad of Dermatol*. 27, 935.

[11] Sperling LC, Lupton GP. Histopathology of nonscarring alopecia. *J Cutan Pathol.* 1995;22:97-114.

[12] Al-refu k & Goodfield M. Basement membrane changes in lichen planopilaris. J Eur Acad Dermatol. 2009. 23 (11), 1289-93.

[13] McDonagh AJG, Messenger AG. The pathogenesis of alopecia areata. Dermatol Clin. 1996;14:661-670.

[14] Elston DM, McCollough ML, Bergfeld WF, Liranzo MO, Heibel M. Eosinophils in fibrous tracts and near hair bulbs: a helpful diagnostic feature of alopecia areata. *J Am Acad Dermatol.* 1997;37:101-106.

[15] David A. Histopathologic Features of Alopecia Areata. Arch Dermatol. 2003;139:1555-1559.

[16] Whiting DA. Diagnostic and predictive value of horizontal sections of scalp biopsy specimens in male pattern androgenetic alopecia. J. Am. Acad. Dermatol. 1993; 28; 755–763.

[17] Whiting D. Scalp biopsy as a diagnostic and prognostic tool in androgenic alopecia. Dermatol. Ther. 1998; 8; 24–33.

Chapter 3

Skin Biopsy Diagnosis of Langerhans Cell Neoplasms

Olga L. Bohn, Julie Teruya-Feldstein and
Sergio Sanchez-Sosa

Additional information is available at the end of the chapter

http://dx.doi.org/10.5772/55893

1. Introduction

This chapter reviews the clinical presentation, histopathology, immunoprofile and molecular features of Langerhans cell neoplasms of the skin including Langerhans cell histiocytosis (LCH) and its malignant counterpart, Langerhans cell sarcoma (LCS). Biopsy of the skin is a useful method to confirm LCH/LCS diagnosis, as cutaneous involvement is seen in more than 50% cases. Skin can be the only presenting site of LCH, but it is usually seen as an integral part of multisystemic disease involvement.

Langerhans cells (LC) are bone marrow-derived antigen presenting cells [1]. Although LC, dendritic cells and monocytic/histiocytic cells share a common multipotential progenitor cells that reside in the bone marrow, to the date, myeloid derived macrophages and dendritic cells constitute divergent lines of differentiation from bone marrow precursors [2]. However, recent evidence demonstrates that LC can be generated from lymphoid-committed $CD4^{low}$ precursors, suggesting the role of lineage plasticity/ trans-differentiation and clonal infidelity [3-4].

LC can be found in the epidermis and mucosal lining of multiple organs including cervix, vagina, stomach and esophagus. The specific immunophenotypic profile is helpful distinguishing LCs, as they can express CD1a and langerin (CD207); in addition the detection of Birbeck granules, seen in both pathological and resting LC is a prominent feature [5].

LCH encompasses a spectrum of disease characterized by an uncontrolled proliferation of LC [5]. The etiology of LCH/LCS is unknown in most cases, and there is not clear understanding of the pathogenesis. Although LCH is believed to be a clonal proliferation of LC [2, 6], the exact nature is controversial, as pulmonary LCH is thought to be a reactive/inflammatory disorder rather than a neoplastic process, and spontaneous remissions have been documented [7-8]. In a recent study of well characterized LCH cases, 30% had clonal immunoglobulin heavy chain (IGH@), immunoglobulin kappa light chain (IGK@) or T-cell receptor gamma (TCRG@) gene rearrangements, suggesting a close relationship between LCH and lymphoid lineage [3]. Additional data that suggests LCH is in fact a clonal disease is the presence of specific mutations such as BRAF V600E, which have been found in up to 76% of tumors in children <10 years of age [7, 9].

2. Langerhans cell histiocytosis

2.1. Clinical presentation

LCH can affect a wide range of patients, including neonates, young children and adults. In children younger than 2 years of age, cutaneous involvement is the most common presentation [10]. In neonates and young infants, skin is frequently involved, as solitary or multiple papules or nodules with ulceration or necrosis. Patients usually present with dermatitis-like lesions that involves scalp, trunk, intertriginous skin folds and perineum with brownish/whitish papules covered with scales and crust [11]. In neonates, eruptions may affect most of the body surface. In contrast, in adults, LCH with initial presentation occurring in the skin is unusual [12].

LCH can be localized, multifocal or multisystemic. Systemic disease can involve organs such as bone marrow, liver, central nervous system, gastrointestinal tract, lungs and spleen. Systemic forms include Letterer-Siwe disease (with skin, lymph node and visceral involvement) and Hand-Schuller-Christian syndrome (in young children).

Congenital disease is rare and often clinically benign, presented in the form of reticulohistiocytosis (Hashimoto-Pritzker disease) as a self-healing or regressive form of the disease. Congenital disease usually presents at birth or in the first few weeks of life as a widespread cutaneous eruption of red-brown nodules that resolves spontaneously [10, 13], although it can rarely be associated with multiorgan involvement [10, 14].

2.2. Histopathology

Recognition of morphologic and immunohistochemical features is essential to establish both the diagnosis and the LC origin. The skin shows a predominant diffuse papillary dermal infiltrate composed of large cells with lobulated, eccentric grooved nuclei with "coffee-bean shape" appearance and inconspicuous nucleoli. The epidermis may be ulcerated and epidermotropism is commonly seen (FIGURE 1).

A variable polymorphic infiltrate of eosinophils, lymphocytes, plasma cells and neutrophils is usually admixed with neoplastic cells. Eosinophils are often but not invariably present, and sometimes can be quite numerous, masking LC (FIGURE 2). Mitotic activity may be brisk. In some cases, LC may resemble histiocytes or Touton cells. Sometimes, a granulomatous reaction with histiocytic infiltrate can be identified.

http://dx.doi.org/10.5772/55893

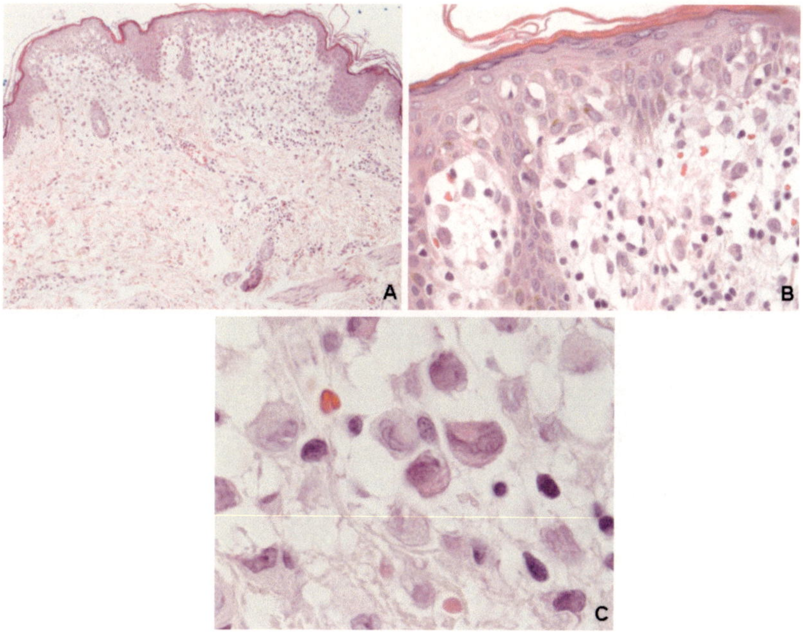

Figure 1. Histological features of Langerhans cell histiocytosis (LCH). A and B. Skin shows dermal infiltrate with epidermotrophism. C. Cells with grooved nuclei.

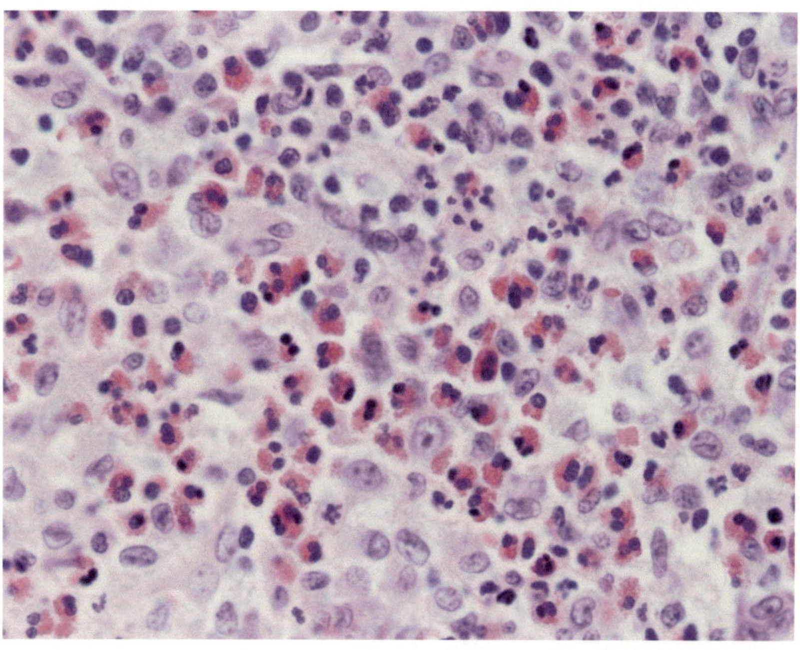

Figure 2. Histological features of Langerhans Cell Histiocytosis (LCH). Skin with inflammatory infiltrate composed of Langerhans cells admixed with abundant eosinophils and neutrophils.

2.3. Immunoprofile and electron microscopy

Identification of LC may be done by routine hematoxylyn-eosin alone. However, confirmation requires positive staining for CD1a, S100 and langerin (CD207) (FIGURE 3), with variable expression of CD68 and usually absence of CD163 stain.

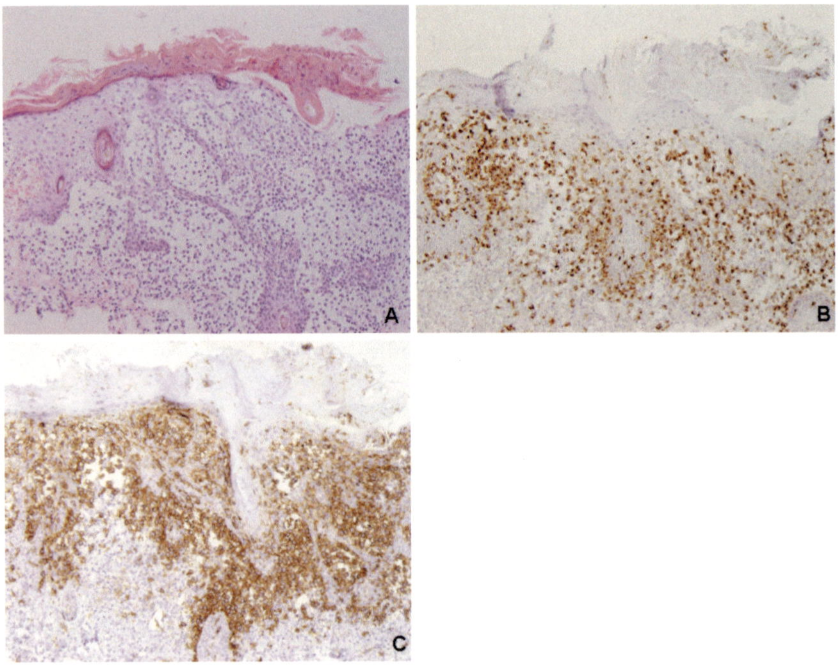

Figure 3. Histological features and immunophenotypic profile of Langerhans Cell Histiocytosis (LCH). A. Skin with dermal infiltrate and epidermotrophism. B. Langerin immunostain (CD207) highlights neoplastic Langerhans Cells (LC). C. LC are positive for CD1a.

A novel antibody, JL1, has been described as a specific marker in LCH. Interestingly, LC in the epidermis of normal skin express langerin but not JL1; however both antibodies are expressed in inflamed skin [5]. In addition, a recent specific antibody to detect BRAFV600E mutation in LCH by immunohistochemistry is identified that can be used for routine screening [15]. E-cadherin expression has been reported as well (FIGURE 4). Electron microscopy can be used to demonstrate intracytoplasmic Birbeck granules of approximately 300 nm with a tennis-racket shape.

2.4. Differential diagnosis

Related and unrelated histiocytic disorders and benign LC proliferations lead to diagnostic pitfalls in LCH. Localized LC proliferations are seen in a vast number of skin conditions that may be reactive, but are often neoplastic. Similarly, histiocytic infiltrates in the dermis are very common, and appear in response to inflammatory conditions, infections and neoplasms.

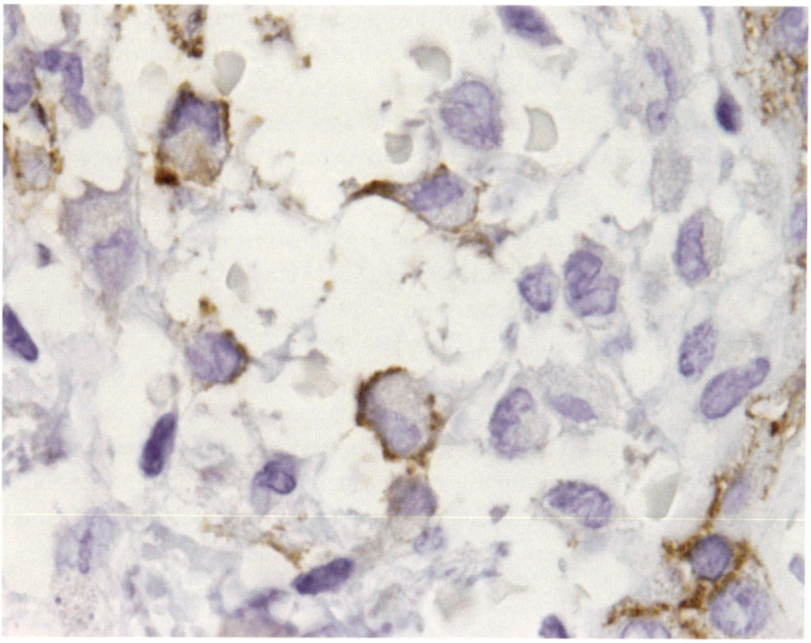

Figure 4. Immunoprofile of Langerhans Cell Histiocytosis. E-cadherin is positive in scattered LC.

LC microabscesses can sometimes be seen in the epidermis of spongiotic dermatitides and lichenoid dermatitis. LC are usually seen as small to large collection of pale staining/mononuclear cells, positive for CD1a and S100. These aggregates can mimic Pautrier's microabscessess in mycosis fungoides [16].

In children with eczematous eruptions and histiocytic infiltrates, langerhans cell hyperplasia (LCHP) has to be ruled out. LCHP can mimic LCH and has been reported in cases of human scabies, arthropod bite reaction, contact dermatitis and pytiriasis lichenoides and usually cells express CD1a and S100 [17-20]. The increased in LC in the dermis can be explained by the antigenic stimulation and cutaneous trauma that produce LC migration into the skin, especially when occurs in perivascular areas. Therefore, the clinical context in which the lesion or proliferation arises is important in the differential diagnosis.

Likewise, reactive histiocytosis in the skin can be seen secondary to foreign body reactions to implants and polarizable material is often identified [21]. LC can also mimic dermal histiocytes found in inflammatory and infectious conditions (mycobacteria, fungal and parasitic processes), thus clinicopathologic correlation, immunostains and appropriate special stain can be helpful in the differential. Eosinophils, a common finding in LCH can also be seen in a variable number of conditions such as drug eruptions, urticaria and wells syndrome.

Furthermore, a group of conditions named as non-Langerhans cells histiocytosis (N-LCH) can mimic LCH. These entities are characterized by accumulation of histiocytes and immunohistochemistry is a useful adjuvant for the distinction; some of them will be describe in the following pages [22].

Rosai-Dorfman disease (RDD) is a self-limiting histio-proliferative disorder that can compromise almost any organ, and occasionally involves the skin [23]. Cutaneous RDD is characterized by the presence of a dense infiltrate of foamy histiocytes with emperipolesis surrounded by a background of lymphocytes, plasma cells and neutrophils. Occasionally, eosinophils can be increased [24]. Histiocytic cells in RDD usually express CD68 and S100 and lack of CD1a staining.

The Juvenile Xantogranuloma (JXG) family is a spectrum of conditions characterized by expression of factor XIIIa, CD68, CD163, fascin and CD14 but lack immunoexpression for CD1a and S100 [22, 24]. The clinical setting is useful to differentiate the entities. JXG is a common member of this family. JXG presents as a solitary skin lesion, most commonly seen throughout the first two decades of life, although some cases have been described in extracutaneous sites. JXG is characterized by circumscribed dermal nodules composed of true foamy histiocytes and Touton giant cells. Touton giant cells are seen in the majority of cases, and show a wreath of nuclei around a homogenous eosinophilic cytoplasm and xanthomatous periphery (FIGURE 5) [22, 25]. JXG has been reported associated with neurofibromatosis type 1, hemophagocytic lymphohistiocytosis and juvenile myelomonocytic chronic leukemia [26-27].

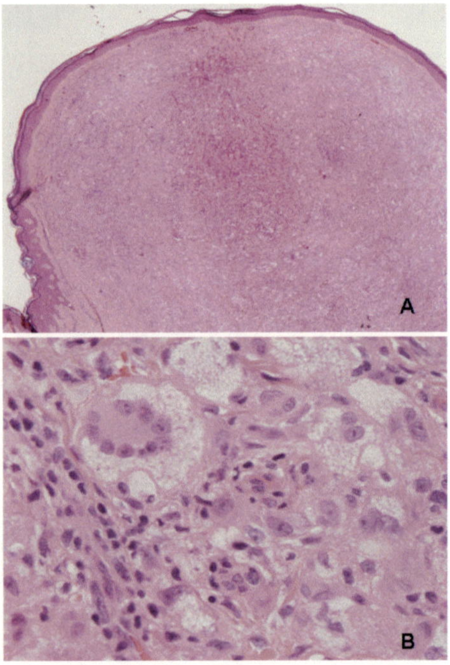

Figure 5. Juvenile Xantogranuloma (JXG). A. Dome shape lesion with dermal infiltrate. B. Touton giant cells in JXG.

Erdheim-Chester disease (ECD) may also be confused by LCH. ECD is a systemic disease which usually presents with lung and symmetrical long bony lesions. It can also involve the skin and clinically appears with pruritic rash, xanthelasma and eyelid xanthomas, in a background of normal lipid profile [28]. ECD displays collections of enlarged histiocytes with clear cytoplasm. ECD can be differentiated from LCH by immunohistochemical studies; ECD cells usually express CD68, CD163, fascin, while negative for S100, langerin and CD1a. Birbeck granules are absent [22].

Finally, a hybrid entity, indeterminate cell histiocytosis (immature dendritic cells) is an uncommon disease with features between LCH and N-LCH. Although it shows immunophenotypic similarities with LCH such as CD1a positivity and variable expression of S100 and CD68, lacks of Birbeck granules by electron microscopy.

Malignant neoplasms such as histiocytic sarcoma (HS), myelomonocytic leukemia, anaplastic large cell lymphoma and mast cell proliferations should also be considered into the differential diagnosis [24, 29]. HS is a malignant proliferation of mature histiocytes. Skin presentation is often seen, although multisystemic involvement is a frequent feature. Histologically, HS show cytologic atypia, pleomorphism and mitotic activity; the immunophenotypic profile demonstrates that the malignant cells are usually positive for CD68, CD163, CD14, CD4, CD11c and lysozyme. Birbeck granules are not seen [30].

Interestingly, cases of LCH have been found in association with malignancy including solid tumors and hematologic neoplasms [31-32]. In a recent study, adult patients with LCH presenting in the skin have shown an increased risk of a second hematological malignancy [12]. They can present with a solitary papule/nodule or multiple reddish-brown papules. The literature includes reports of LCH and non-Hodgkin lymphoma, Hodgkin lymphoma, acute lymphoblastic leukemia [33] and acute myeloid leukemia (AML) [31, 34-38]. One of the current theories that could explain the association between LCH and AML relates to trans-differentiation of hematopoietic lineages as LC, dendritic cells, and monocytic/histiocytic cells share common multipotential progenitor cells that reside in the bone marrow [39-42]. These cases suggest a clonal relation between the two neoplastic diseases and support the theories of lineage plasticity in mature and immature lymphoid tumors.

2.5. Prognosis

LCH is a heterogeneous disease with different outcomes including self healing-limited and life-threatening or fatal disease [14]. Clinical staging is a prognostic marker in neonates and infants [14, 43]. Unifocal/localized disease has a good prognosis and long term survival. In contrast, the clinical course and the prognosis of multifocal and multisystemic disease are difficult to predict. When disseminated disease is present at the time of diagnosis, the disease is usually associated with poor outcome [14, 43]. Therefore, identification of specific biomarkers is needed in order to determine who will have limited disease and who will benefit from systemic therapy.

Using OncoMap, the activating mutation BRAF V600E mutation has been recently identified as a recurrent molecular genetic aberration in LCH, however, its clinical significance is still unknown [7, 9, 14]. BRAF V600E mutations have been identified in LCH and ECD, however, they have not seen in RDD and JXG [44]. Interestingly, inhibition of BRAF V600E may be used in the near future as a therapeutic target for LCH similar to what is being done for melanoma, gliomas and hairy cell leukemia. Patients with positive mutation status and protein expression by screening may be allowed for protocol or clinical trial entry with use of Zelboraf (vemurafinib), an FDA approved therapy. Recently, a variant BRAF V600D mutation has been reported in congenital, benign, self-regressive LCH [14]. E-cadherin expression was found as a marker of good prognosis and limited disease, however, the results have not been validated in separated studies [10, 45]. The role of Ki67 as a prognostic marker is limited. One of the most common abnormalities seen in LCH is TP53 over-expression (FIGURE 6); however, TP53 mutations have not been identified [7, 9, 46].

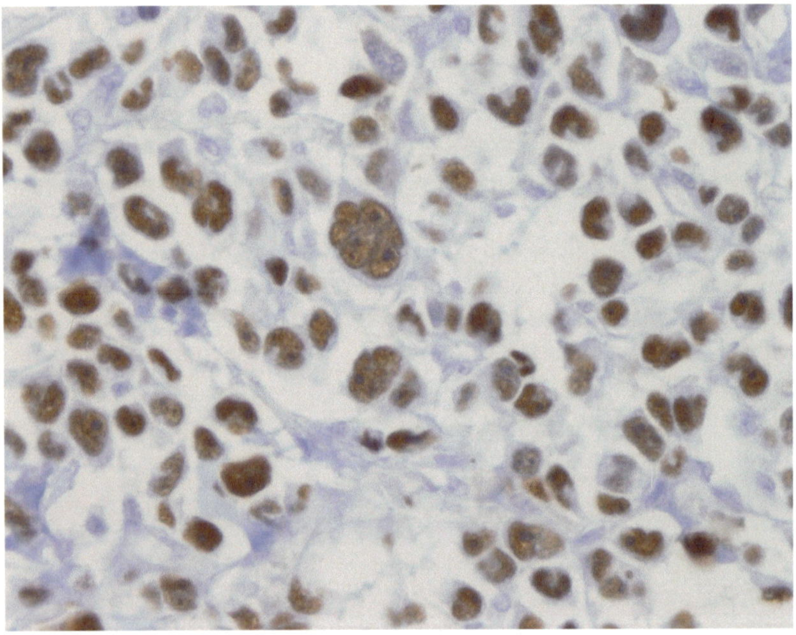

Figure 6. TP53 over-expression in Langerhans Cell Histiocytosis (LCH)

2.6. Treatment

Patients require complete clinical history, physical examination, and a comprehensive laboratory and radiographic evaluation [47]. The Histiocyte Society recommends that in order to determine the adequate research protocol, patients should be stratified based upon extension of the disease (unifocal, multifocal/multysistemic), involvement of risk organs (hemato-lymphoid including spleen and liver) and central nervous system risk lesions [48-49]. Patients with unifocal disease limited to the skin require follow up-and usually no additional treatment is necessary as spontaneous regression may occur. Topical therapy with steroids or PUVA may be used [48]. In cases of multiorgan/multisystemic involvement, the treatment is controversial as those patients have a variable clinical course; it includes systemic chemotherapy with assessment of clinical response after the first 6 weeks of treatment. Monoclonal antibodies are under research. In one large study, Vinblastine with or without prednisolone was the most common chemotherapy regimen, and the overall survival and event free survival rates were 84% and 51.5%, respectively with a medium follow-up time of 8 years [50]. The LCHIII treatment protocol is a common strategy used in patients with multiorgan involvement [51]. Targeted therapy with vemurafenib, an inhibitor of mutated BRAF, has been used in few patients with LCH harboring BRAF V600E mutation [52].

3. Langerhans cell sarcoma

3.1. Clinical presentation

Thirty one cases of LCS have been reported to date [53]. Skin can be a single site involved by LCS or can be seen as part of widespread disease. Cutaneous involvement is present in more than half of cases. Multiorgan involvement includes lymph node, lungs, liver, spleen and bone. Skin biopsy is an accessible and a useful way to demonstrate malignant LC. LCS occurs in all age groups with a male:female ratio 1:1. LCS can appear as an increasingly progressive malignant disease followed by multiple LCH recurrences, *de novo* and with underlying myeloproliferative disease [53-55]. *De novo* or primary LCS has been reported exclusively in adults, without previous evidence of LCH. In a recent publication, a case of trans-differentiation of acute B-lymphoblastic leukemia into a LCS has been documented, as both show identical IGH@ gene rearrangements [54].

3.2. Histopathology

Skin biopsy usually shows an infiltrative and poorly defined high grade malignant neoplasm composed of large cells with grooved nuclei, granular chromatin, prominent nucleoli and high mitotic rate. Although inflammatory infiltrate can be present and abundant, especially if there is associated necrosis, eosinophils are usually scattered. Epidermis can be ulcerated and epidermotropism is seen [2, 55]. (FIGURE 7)

3.3. Immunoprofile and electron microscopy

Malignant LC are usually positive for CD1a, S100 and Langerin (CD207) (FIGURE 8). There is lack of reactivity for T and B cell antigens. Neoplastic cells have a high proliferative Ki67 index and overexpress p53. CD56 /neural cell adhesion molecule (NCAM) positivity has been found expressed in LCS [56]. A broad panel of immunohistochemical stains is used to confirm LC due to the atypical features of the neoplasm, and electron microscopy is usually performed for identification of intracytoplasmic Birbeck granules.

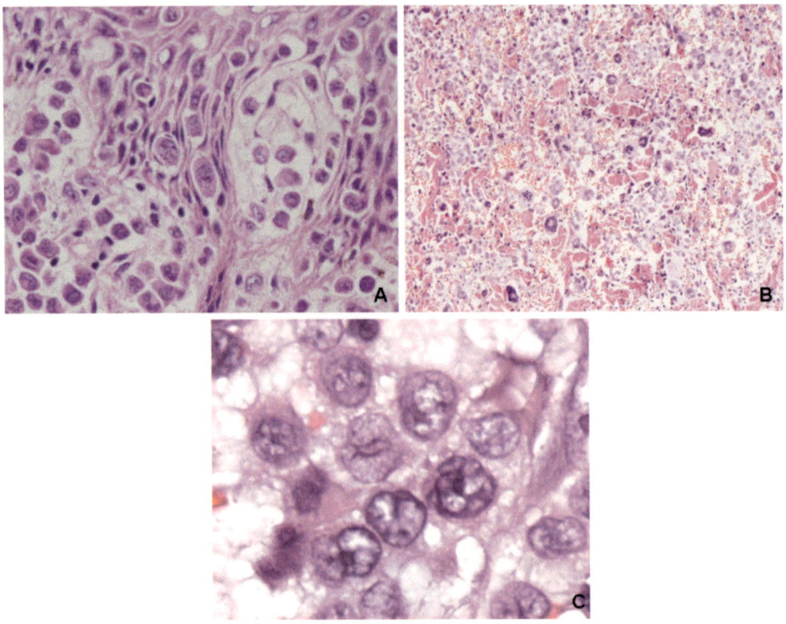

Figure 7. Histological appearance of Langerhans Cell Sarcoma (LCS). A. Dermal infiltrate of large atypical cells with epidermotrophism. B. Bizarre and pleomorphic cells with abundant mitotic figures and lack of cohesiveness. C. Detailed figure of LCS cells with prominent intranuclear inclusions.

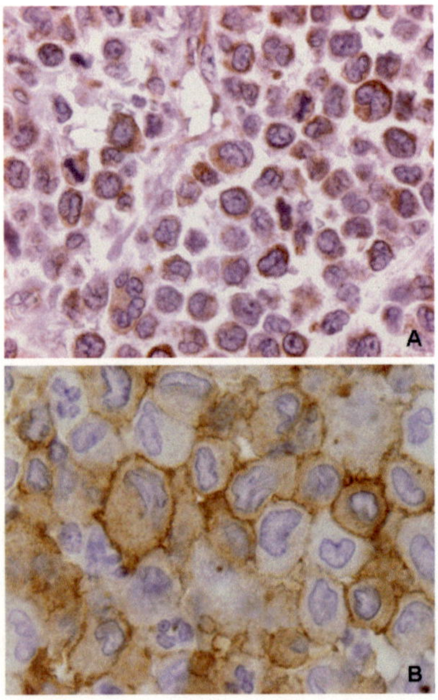

Figure 8. Immunoprofile of Langerhans Cell Sarcoma (LCS). A. Langerin (CD207) expression in cells with malignant features. Numerous mitotic figures are identified. B. Malignant cells retain CD1a expression.

3.4. Differential diagnosis

Because of the marked pleomorphism and cytologic atypia, hematologic and nonhematologic entities must be considered in the differential diagnosis including malignant melanoma, carcinoma, mesenchymal malignant neoplasms and lymphomas with anaplastic features. Pleomorphic large cells may be mistaken for malignant melanoma, which shares S100 positivity but also expresses other melanocytic markers. LCS comprises cells with bizarre pleomorphic nuclei and abundant cytoplasm mimicking hematolymphoid neoplasms including anaplastic large cell lymphoma, anaplastic diffuse large B-cell lymphoma, plasma cell neoplasm with anaplastic features, lymphomatoid papulosis, peripheral T cell lymphoma and myeloid sarcoma (FIGURE 9) (TABLE 1) [55]. In those cases, immunohistochemical and molecular features are useful to distinguish the cell of origin.

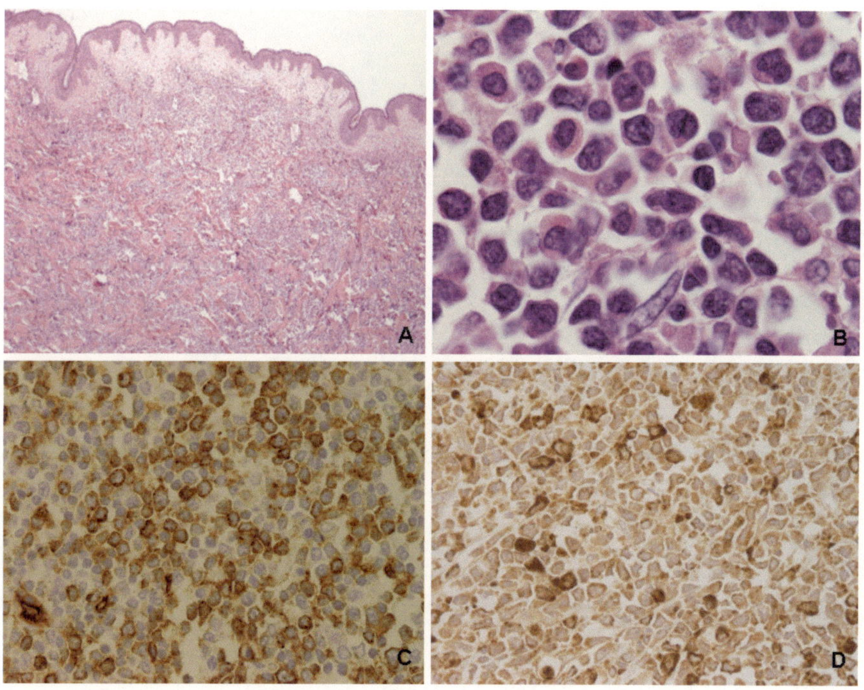

Figure 9. Myeloid Sarcoma. A. Skin shows a diffuse dermal infiltrate composed of malignant cells. B. Features of neoplastic cells with promyelocytic differentiation. C. CD34 stain is positive in the majority of cells. D. Myeloperoxidase (MPO) positivity in tumor cells.

DIFFERENTIAL DIAGNOSIS	Immunohistochemical marker
Melanoma	S100+, Melan A+, HMB45+
Anaplastic large cell lymphoma	CD30+, ALK+/-, EMA+, CD3-/+, CD43+
Histiocytic Sarcoma	CD68+, CD163+, CD14+, CD4+, lysozyme, S100+/-
Follicular Dendritic Cell Sarcoma	CD21+, CD23+, CD35+, CD68+/-, S100+/-, Clusterin+, CD45+/-
Interdigitating Dendritic Cell Sarcoma	S100+, CD21-, CD35-, CD1a-, fascin +, CD68-/+
Myeloid Sarcoma	CD34+, CD117+, MPO+, CD68+, lysozyme+

Table 1. Langerhans Cell Sarcoma (LCS) - Differential Diagnosis

3.5. Prognosis and treatment

Currently, no specific marker has demonstrated to predict prognosis in LCS. In a study, CD56 expression was associated to poor prognosis and the results have not been validated in a different set of patients [56]. Despite combination chemotherapy/radiotherapy and surgery, LCS is an aggressive high grade malignancy with poor prognosis, frequent recurrences and short survival, usually resulting in death within 1 year [2, 53, 55].

Author details

Olga L. Bohn[1], Julie Teruya-Feldstein[1] and Sergio Sanchez-Sosa[2]

*Address all correspondence to: bohno@mskcc.org

1 Department of Pathology, Memorial Sloan-Kettering Cancer Center, New York, NY, USA

2 Department of Pathology, Hospital Angeles, Puebla, Mexico

References

[1] Romani, N, Clausen, B. E, & Stoitzner, P. Langerhans cells and more: langerin-expressing dendritic cell subsets in the skin. Immunol Rev. (2010). Mar;, 234(1), 120-41.

[2] Jaffe, R W. L, & Facchetti, F. Tumors derived from Langerhans cells. 4th Edition ed. Swerlow SH CE, Harris NL, Jaffe ES, Pileri SA, Stein H, Thiele J, Vardiman JW, editor. Lyon: International Agency for Research on Cancer; (2008).

[3] Chen, W, Wang, J, Wang, E, Lu, Y, Lau, S. K, Weiss, L. M, et al. Detection of clonal lymphoid receptor gene rearrangements in langerhans cell histiocytosis. Am J Surg Pathol. (2010). Jul;, 34(7), 1049-57.

[4] Anjuere, F. del Hoyo GM, Martin P, Ardavin C. Langerhans cells develop from a lymphoid-committed precursor. Blood. (2000). Sep 1;, 96(5), 1633-7.

[5] Park, H. J, Jeon, Y. K, Lee, A. H, Oh, Y. H, Park, S. H, & Jung, K. C. Use of the JL1 epitope, which encompasses the nonglycosylation site of CD43, as a marker of immature/neoplastic Langerhans cells. Am J Surg Pathol. (2012). Aug;, 36(8), 1150-7.

[6] Willman, C. L, Busque, L, Griffith, B. B, Favara, B. E, Mcclain, K. L, Duncan, M. H, et al. Langerhans'-cell histiocytosis (histiocytosis X)--a clonal proliferative disease. N Engl J Med. (1994). Jul 21;, 331(3), 154-60.

[7] Badalian-very, G, Vergilio, J. A, & Degar, B. A. MacConaill LE, Brandner B, Calicchio ML, et al. Recurrent BRAF mutations in Langerhans cell histiocytosis. Blood. (2010). Sep 16;, 116(11), 1919-23.

[8] Mcelligott, J, Mcmichael, A, Sangueza, O. P, Anthony, E, Rose, D, & Mclean, T. W. Spontaneous regression of langerhans cell histiocytosis in a neonate with multiple bony lesions. J Pediatr Hematol Oncol. (2008). Jan;, 30(1), 85-6.

[9] Badalian-very, G, Vergilio, J. A, Degar, B. A, Rodriguez-galindo, C, & Rollins, B. J. Recent advances in the understanding of Langerhans cell histiocytosis. Br J Haematol. (2012). Jan;, 156(2), 163-72.

[10] Kapur, P, Erickson, C, Rakheja, D, Carder, K. R, & Hoang, M. P. Congenital self-healing reticulohistiocytosis (Hashimoto-Pritzker disease): ten-year experience at Dallas Children's Medical Center. J Am Acad Dermatol. (2007). Feb;, 56(2), 290-4.

[11] Elder, D. E E. R, Johnson, B, Ioffreda, M, Miller, J, & Miller, O. F. editor. Lever's Histopathology of the skin. 9th edition ed. Philadelphia: Lippincott Williams & Wilkins; (2004).

[12] Edelbroek, J. R, Vermeer, M. H, Jansen, P. M, Stoof, T. J, Van Der Linden, M. M, Horvath, B, et al. Langerhans cell histiocytosis first presenting in the skin in adults: frequent association with a second hematological malignancy. Br J Dermatol. (2012). Jul 27.

[13] Hashimoto, K, & Pritzker, M. S. Electron microscopic study of reticulohistiocytoma. An unusual case of congenital, self-healing reticulohistiocytosis. Arch Dermatol. (1973). Feb;, 107(2), 263-70.

[14] Kansal, R, Quintanilla-martinez, L, Datta, V, Lopategui, J, Garshfield, G, & Nathwani, B. N. Identification of the mutation in Exon 15 of the BRAF oncogene in congenital, benign langerhans cell histiocytosis. Genes Chromosomes Cancer. (2012). Sep 21., 600D

[15] Sahm, F, Capper, D, Preusser, M, Meyer, J, Stenzinger, A, Lasitschka, F, et al. BRAFV600E mutant protein is expressed in cells of variable maturation in Langerhans cell histiocytosis. Blood. (2012). Sep 20;120(12):e, 28-34.

[16] Candiago, E, Marocolo, D, Manganoni, M. A, Leali, C, & Facchetti, F. Nonlymphoid intraepidermal mononuclear cell collections (pseudo-Pautrier abscesses): a morphologic and immunophenotypical characterization. Am J Dermatopathol. (2000). Feb;, 22(1), 1-6.

[17] Bhattacharjee, P, & Glusac, E. J. Langerhans cell hyperplasia in scabies: a mimic of Langerhans cell histiocytosis. J Cutan Pathol. (2007). Sep;, 34(9), 716-20.

[18] Drut, R, Peral, C. G, Garone, A, & Rositto, A. Langerhans cell hyperplasia of the skin mimicking Langerhans cell histiocytosis: a report of two cases in children not associated with scabies. Fetal Pediatr Pathol. (2010). , 29(4), 231-8.

[19] Burch, J. M, Krol, A, & Weston, W. L. Sarcoptes scabiei infestation misdiagnosed and treated as Langerhans cell histiocytosis. Pediatr Dermatol. (2004). Jan-Feb;, 21(1), 58-62.

[20] Kim, S. H, Kim, D. H, & Lee, K. G. Prominent Langerhans' cell migration in the arthropod bite reactions simulating Langerhans' cell histiocytosis. J Cutan Pathol. (2007). Dec;, 34(12), 899-902.

[21] Miller, D. D, Yaar, R, Posnik, O, Karolow, W, & Mahalingam, M. Reactive granular histiocytosis secondary to arthroplasty prosthesis: a novel reaction pattern. J Cutan Pathol. (2012). May;, 39(5), 558-61.

[22] Weitzman, S, & Jaffe, R. Uncommon histiocytic disorders: the non-Langerhans cell histiocytoses. Pediatr Blood Cancer. (2005). Sep;, 45(3), 256-64.

[23] Rosai, J, & Dorfman, R. F. Sinus histiocytosis with massive lymphadenopathy. A newly recognized benign clinicopathological entity. Arch Pathol. (1969). Jan;, 87(1), 63-70.

[24] Cangelosi, J. J, Prieto, V. G, & Ivan, D. Cutaneous Rosai-Dorfman disease with increased number of eosinophils: coincidence or histologic variant? Arch Pathol Lab Med. (2011). Dec;, 135(12), 1597-600.

[25] Dehner, L. P. Juvenile xanthogranulomas in the first two decades of life: a clinicopathologic study of 174 cases with cutaneous and extracutaneous manifestations. Am J Surg Pathol. (2003). May;, 27(5), 579-93.

[26] Arachchillage, D. R, Carr, T. F, Kerr, B, Hawkins, K, Kelsey, A, Judge, M, et al. Juvenile myelomonocytic leukemia presenting with features of neonatal hemophagocytic lymphohistiocytosis and cutaneous juvenile xanthogranulomata and successfully treated with allogeneic hemopoietic stem cell transplant. J Pediatr Hematol Oncol. (2010). Mar;, 32(2), 152-5.

[27] Raygada, M, Arthur, D. C, Wayne, A. S, Rennert, O. M, Toretsky, J. A, & Stratakis, C. A. Juvenile xanthogranuloma in a child with previously unsuspected neurofibromatosis type 1 and juvenile myelomonocytic leukemia. Pediatr Blood Cancer. (2010). Jan;, 54(1), 173-5.

[28] Veyssier-belot, C, Cacoub, P, Caparros-lefebvre, D, Wechsler, J, Brun, B, Remy, M, et al. Erdheim-Chester disease. Clinical and radiologic characteristics of 59 cases. Medicine (Baltimore). (1996). May;, 75(3), 157-69.

[29] Huang, S. C, Chang, C. L, Huang, C. H, & Chang, C. C. Histiocytic sarcoma- a case with evenly distributed multinucleated giant cells. Pathol Res Pract. (2007). , 203(9), 683-9.

[30] Chang, K. L W. L. editor. Other Histiocytic and Dendritic Cell Neoplasms. 1st ed ed. Philadelphia, PA: Saunders/Elsevier; (2011).

[31] Ghosn, M. G, Haddad, A. C, Nassar, M. N, Abadjian, G. A, El Karak, F. R, & Aftimos, P. G. Acute myeloid leukemia and Langerhans' cell histiocytosis: multiple theories for an unusual presentation. Leuk Res. (2010). Mar;, 34(3), 406-8.

[32] Egeler, R. M, Neglia, J. P, Puccetti, D. M, Brennan, C. A, & Nesbit, M. E. Association of Langerhans cell histiocytosis with malignant neoplasms. Cancer. (1993). Feb 1;, 71(3), 865-73.

[33] Castro, E. C, Blazquez, C, Boyd, J, Correa, H, De Chadarevian, J. P, Felgar, R. E, et al. Clinicopathologic features of histiocytic lesions following ALL, with a review of the literature. Pediatr Dev Pathol. (2010). May-Jun;, 13(3), 225-37.

[34] Egeler, R. M, Neglia, J. P, Arico, M, Favara, B. E, Heitger, A, & Nesbit, M. E. Acute leukemia in association with Langerhans cell histiocytosis. Med Pediatr Oncol. (1994). , 23(2), 81-5.

[35] Arico, M, Comelli, A, Bossi, G, Raiteri, E, Piombo, M, & Egeler, R. M. Langerhans cell histiocytosis and acute leukemia: unusual association in two cases. Med Pediatr Oncol. (1993). , 21(4), 271-3.

[36] Haupt, R, Comelli, A, Rosanda, C, Sessarego, M, & De Bernardi, B. Acute myeloid leukemia after single-agent treatment with etoposide for Langerhans' cell histiocytosis of bone. Am J Pediatr Hematol Oncol. (1993). May;, 15(2), 255-7.

[37] Matsuzaki, A, Inamitsu, T, Watanabe, T, Ohga, S, Ishii, E, Nagotoshi, Y, et al. Acute promyelocytic leukaemia in a patient treated with etoposide for Langerhans cell histiocytosis. Br J Haematol. (1994). Apr;, 86(4), 887-9.

[38] Stine, K. C, Saylors, R. L, Sawyer, J. R, & Becton, D. L. Secondary acute myelogenous leukemia following safe exposure to etoposide. J Clin Oncol. (1997). Apr;, 15(4), 1583-6.

[39] Misery, L, Guyotat, D, & Cambazard, F. Association of Langerhans-cell histiocytosis and acute monocytic leukemia]. Ann Dermatol Venereol. (1998). Oct;, 125(10), 732-3.

[40] Misery, L, Campos, L, Dezutter-dambuyant, C, Guyotat, D, Treille, D, Schmitt, D, et al. CD1-reactive leukemic cells in bone marrow: presence of Langerhans cell marker on leukemic monocytic cells. Eur J Haematol. (1992). Jan;, 48(1), 27-32.

[41] Feldman, A. L, Arber, D. A, Pittaluga, S, Martinez, A, Burke, J. S, Raffeld, M, et al. Clonally related follicular lymphomas and histiocytic/dendritic cell sarcomas: evidence for transdifferentiation of the follicular lymphoma clone. Blood. (2008). Jun 15;, 111(12), 5433-9.

[42] Akashi, K, Traver, D, Miyamoto, T, & Weissman, I. L. A clonogenic common myeloid progenitor that gives rise to all myeloid lineages. Nature. (2000). Mar 9;, 404(6774), 193-7.

[43] Jaffe, R. Is there a role for histopathology in predicting the clinical outcome in congenital and infant Langerhans cell disease? Pediatr Blood Cancer. (2009). Dec;, 53(6), 924-5.

[44] Haroche, J, Charlotte, F, Arnaud, L, Von Deimling, A, Helias-rodzewicz, Z, Hervier, B, et al. High prevalence of BRAF mutations in Erdheim-Chester disease but not in other non-Langerhans cell histiocytoses. Blood. (2012). Sep 27;120(13):2700-3., 600E

[45] Geissmann, F, Emile, J. F, Andry, P, Thomas, C, Fraitag, S, De Prost, Y, et al. Lack of expression of E-cadherin is associated with dissemination of Langerhans' cell histiocytosis and poor outcome. J Pathol. (1997). Mar;, 181(3), 301-4.

[46] da Costa CESzuhai K, van Eijk R, Hoogeboom M, Sciot R, Mertens F, et al. No genomic aberrations in Langerhans cell histiocytosis as assessed by diverse molecular technologies. Genes Chromosomes Cancer. (2009). Mar;, 48(3), 239-49.

[47] Haupt, R, Minkov, M, Astigarraga, I, Schafer, E, Nanduri, V, Jubran, R, et al. Langerhans cell histiocytosis (LCH): Guidelines for diagnosis, clinical work-up, and treatment for patients till the age of 18 years. Pediatr Blood Cancer. (2013). Feb;, 60(2), 175-84.

[48] Satter, E. K, & High, W. A. Langerhans cell histiocytosis: a review of the current recommendations of the Histiocyte Society. Pediatr Dermatol. (2008). May-Jun;, 25(3), 291-5.

[49] Grois, N, Potschger, U, Prosch, H, Minkov, M, Arico, M, Braier, J, et al. Risk factors for diabetes insipidus in langerhans cell histiocytosis. Pediatr Blood Cancer. (2006). Feb;, 46(2), 228-33.

[50] Yagci, B, Varan, A, Caglar, M, Soylemezoglu, F, Sungur, A, Orhan, D, et al. Langerhans cell histiocytosis: retrospective analysis of 217 cases in a single center. Pediatr Hematol Oncol. (2008). Jun;, 25(5), 399-408.

[51] Satter, E. K. A presumptive case of Kindler syndrome with a new clinical finding. Pediatr Dermatol. (2008). Nov-Dec;, 25(6), 646-8.

[52] Haroche, J, Cohen-aubart, F, Emile, J. F, Arnaud, L, Maksud, P, Charlotte, F, et al. Dramatic efficacy of vemurafenib in both multisystemic and refractory Erdheim-Chester disease and Langerhans cell histiocytosis harboring the BRAF mutation. Blood. (2012). Dec 20., 600E

[53] Sagransky, M. J, Deng, A. C, & Magro, C. M. Primary Cutaneous Langerhans Cell Sarcoma: A report of Four Cases and Review of the Literature. Am J Dermatopathol. (2012). Oct 9.

[54] Ratei, R, Hummel, M, Anagnostopoulos, I, Jahne, D, Arnold, R, Dorken, B, et al. Common clonal origin of an acute B-lymphoblastic leukemia and a Langerhans' cell sarcoma: evidence for hematopoietic plasticity. Haematologica. (2010). Sep;, 95(9), 1461-6.

[55] Bohn, O. L, Ruiz-arguelles, G, Navarro, L, Saldivar, J, & Sanchez-sosa, S. Cutaneous Langerhans cell sarcoma: a case report and review of the literature. Int J Hematol. (2007). Feb;, 85(2), 116-20.

[56] Kawase, T, Hamazaki, M, Ogura, M, Kawase, Y, Murayama, T, Mori, Y, et al. CD56/NCAM-positive Langerhans cell sarcoma: a clinicopathologic study of 4 cases. Int J Hematol. (2005). May;, 81(4), 323-9.

Chapter 4

Severe Cutaneous Adverse Reactions

Suran L. Fernando

Additional information is available at the end of the chapter

http://dx.doi.org/10.5772/54820

1. Introduction

Severe cutaneous adverse reactions (SCARs) are generally induced by drugs and encompass the conditions of Stevens-Johnson syndrome (SJS) and toxic epidermal necrolysis (TEN), drug induced eosinophilia and systemic syndrome (DRESS) also known as drug induced hypersensitivity syndrome (DIHS), and acute generalized exanthematous pustulosis (AGEP). These conditions, although rare, cause significant morbidity and are potentially fatal. It is therefore important for the treating physician to promptly recognize SCARs through the identification of their characteristic clinical features so that the offending drug is promptly withdrawn and supportive and adjunctive therapies are administered. SCARs are accompanied by particular abnormalities on routine laboratory investigations and skin biopsy that enables confirmation of the diagnosis and provision of useful prognostic information. Data bases have been established, predominantly in Europe, since the 1980s to characterize the epidemiology of SCARs including the identification of drugs with the highest relative risk and the latency between the commencement of drug intake and the onset of clinical manifestations. The pathogenesis of the various SCARs involves delayed T cell-mediated inflammation in a genetically predisposed individual and in the case of DIHS, may involve viral factors. The emerging field of the genetic susceptibility to SCARs has raised the important issue of pharmacogenetic screening as a method of predicting an individual's risk of developing SCAR to a certain drug. The treatment of SJS/TEN is dependent on supportive care in a suitable settling such as a Burns Unit and the role of immunomodulatory agents is not well defined and is not robustly supported in the literature by prospective studies. The evidence for the use of immunomodulatory agents and ganciclovir is emerging in the treatment of DIHS/DRESS. AGEP usually has favourable prognosis if the offending drug is withdrawn but a course of corticosteroids may hasten recovery.

1.1. SJS/TEN

Stevens-Johnson Syndrome (SJS), first described in 1922 as an acute mucocutaneous syndrome in two boys, and Toxic Epidermal Necrolysis (TEN), first described as a scalding eruption of the skin in 1956 in four patients, are now considered to lie along the spectrum of epidermal necrolysis. The terminology is based on the extent of epidermal detachment; SJS indicates that there is less than 10% detachment of the body surface area, TEN greater than 30%, and SJS/TEN overlap between 10 and 30%.

The clinical presentation is characterized by a rash featuring target-like lesions, and mucositis involving the ocular, oropharyngeal and genital surfaces. The patient is also systemically unwell with fever and malaise. The EuroSCAR case control study collected 379 cases of SJS/TEN between 1997 and 2001 from 6 countries encompassing over 100 million inhabitants. The estimated incidence is 1-2 per million per year. The drugs associated with the highest relative risk include allopurinol, antibacterial sulphonamides, oxicam non-steroidal anti-inflammatory drugs (NSAIDs), aromatic anticonvulsants (phenytoin, carbamazepine, pheno-barbital), lamotrigine, and nevirapine. The latency between the intake of these high-risk drugs and the onset of clinical manifestations is 1 to 8 weeks. Other factors influencing risk include the presence of other diseases (HIV, malignancy, autoimmune disease, recent radiotherapy, acute infection within the last four weeks) and pharmacokinetic factors (dose of allopurinol commenced at 200-300 mg daily). Recently, genes conferring strong susceptibility to SJS/TEN have been identified, the most prominent of which are HLA-B*1502 and carbamazepine in individuals of Asian ancestry, HLA-A*3101 and carbamazepine in individuals from Northern European ancestry, and HLA-B*5801 and allopurinol in various racial groups. A black box warning has been placed by the Food and Drugs Administration and Health Canada alerting physicians to not only to be aware of the risk of carbamazepine and SJS/TEN in Asians but to also screen at risk individuals for the susceptibility allele. Currently, this strategy has been limited by the lack of availability of cost-effective pharmacogenetic testing methods to the general physician.

The immunopathogenesis of SJS/TEN involves the release of granulysin by CD8 cytotoxic T cells and natural killer cells within the epidermis resulting in apoptosis of keratinocytes. Apoptosis may also result from the degranulation of perforin and granzyme by CD8 cytotoxic T cells and the ligation of Fas on keratinocytes by Fas-ligand (Fas-L). The source of Fas-L is still unclear with CD8 cells and keratinocytes proposed as candidates. Histologically, the resultant widespread apoptosis of keratinocytes results in necrosis of the epidermis and dermoepidermal separation at the level of the stratum spinosum. Direct immunofluorescence of skin biopsies in SJS/TEN is negative differentiating it from autoimmune vesiculobullous diseases.

The diagnosis is made clinically and confirmed histologically. Skin testing is contraindicated given the risk of precipitating a generalized reaction. In vitro tests are currently not widely available and relatively poor sensitivity. Lymphocyte transformation tests that assess the proliferative response of T cells to the drug have a sensitivity of 60-70% and are more likely to be positive if performed within 6 weeks of the onset of the disease. Cytotoxicity assays that determine the extent of degranulation of cytotoxic T cells by flow cytometry or ELISA may prove useful in the future.

The treatment of SJS involves the removal of the offending drug and supportive treatment depending on severity and availability in a burns unit to address the manifestations and complications of acute skin failure including monitoring of fluid-electrolyte balance, provision of enteral or parenteral nutrition, wound care and treatment of sepsis. In addition, supportive care of affected mucosal surfaces is required. This includes aggressive ocular lubrication, topical corticosteroids and topical antibiotics, hygienic mouthwashes and topical oral anaesthetics, and monitoring for urinary retention. Large randomized trials on the benefits of immunomodulatory therapy is lacking but there is sufficient evidence to recommend the administration of intravenous immunoglobulin (IVIg) as it contains anti-FasL antibodies and as a result may halt further epidermal necrosis and hasten re-epithelialization. Cyclosporin due to its effects on cytotoxic T cell depletion has reported to be of benefit in a number of small studies. A number of early studies revealed that systemic corticosteroids may be not be beneficial in the treatment of SJS/TEN and in fact may be harmful by promoting sepsis but these conclusions may have been partly explained by the inadequate doses administered and the delay in initiating treatment. Recent studies have demonstrated benefit in the immediate use of high dose pulse methylprednisolone, especially in reducing the rate of ocular complications. The application of amniotic membranes to the conjunctival surface may also prove beneficial in minimising ocular sequelae such as dry eye, cicatrization and in rare cases, corneal perforation.

The mortality rate of SJS/TEN is high; approximately 10% for SJS and 50% for TEN. A score for the evaluation of TEN (SCORTEN) has proven remarkably accurate in predicting mortality through identification of 6 risk factors; age > 40 years, presence of malignancy, heart rate > 120/min, epidermal detachment > 10%, serum urea > 10 mmol/L (28 mg/dL), serum glucose > 14 mmol/L (252 mg/dL) and serum bicarbonate < 20 mmol/L (20 mEq/L).

2. DIHS/DRESS

DIHS/DRESS is also referred to as hypersensitivity syndrome and when caused by antiepileptic drugs it has been often referred to as anticonvulsant hypersensitivity. The condition is characterised by fever, rash, lymphadenopathy, eosinophilia and/or other leukocyte abnormalities, and internal organ involvement such as hepatitis. Reactivation of human herpes virus (HHV)-6 is also considered by some groups to be an instrumental component of the condition. The rash typically begins as patchy erythematous macules that become confluent and progresses especially if the causative drug is not withdrawn to an erythroderma or exfoliative dermatitis. The syndrome typically develops between 3 weeks and 3 months after the starting therapy and a limited number of drugs appear involved in its causation. They include anticonvulsants (phenytoin, carbamazepine, phenobarbital, lamotrigine, zonisaminde), allopurinol, sulphonamides (dapsone, sulphasalazine), antiretrovirals (abacavir, nevirapine), minocycline, strontium ranelate, and mexilitene. The precise incidence according to the latest case definition will be determined by RegiSCAR study, which comprises data collected from 6 European countries and the JSCAR Japanese registry. The incidence following phenytoin therapy is estimated to be 1 in 1000 to 10000 exposures.

DIHS has a relapsing remitting course lasting several weeks to months despite the withdrawal of the offending drug and this has been postulated to result from the sequential reactivation of herpes viruses analogous to that observed in graft versus host disease. The precise role of HHV-6 in DIHS is unclear. One theory is that HHV-6 triggers DIHS through its reactivation within T cells resulting in HHV-6 stimulated T cells cross-reacting with the culprit drug, following which there is sequential activation of heterologous herpes viruses. The alternative explanation is that drug specific T cells are activated resulting in reactivation of the viral genome and sequential reactivation of herpes viruses.

The histological features of DIHS are relatively non-specific and typically comprise a superficial perivascular lymphocytic infiltrate. As the understanding of the disease mechanisms emerge, novel findings such as granulomatous inflammation have also been identified.

The diagnostic criteria consist of the typical clinical features and laboratory abnormalities. Confirmation of the role of the causative agent by skin testing is contraindicated because of the risk of a generalized reaction. The utility of LTTs is unclear as they are often negative early in the course of disease possibly as a result of regulatory T cell activation. LTTs may become positive after 5-7 weeks as the expanded regulatory T cell population are removed by apoptosis at the end of the immune response.

A prolonged course of oral corticosteroids is required to treat DIHS given the relapsing remitting nature of the condition. The mortality rate is estimated to be 10-20%.

3. AGEP

AGEP is rare with an incidence of 1-5 cases per million per year. The clinical manifestations are characterised by fever and the rapid appearance of disseminated sterile pustules 3-5 days after the commencement of treatment. It is accompanied by a marked neutrophilia. Mucous membranes are not typically involved. The drugs conferring the highest risk of AGEP according to the EuroSCAR study are aminopenicillins, pristinamycin, hydroxychloroquine, antibacterial sulphonamides, terbinafine and diltiazem. The pathogenesis of AGEP involves the initial influx of CD8 cytotoxic T cells resulting in apoptosis of keratinocytes and formation of vesicles. Then CXCL-8 producing CD4 cells enter the epidermis resulting in neutrophil mediated inflammation and formation of pustules. As a result the histology reveals intraepidermal usually subcorneal pustules and an accompanying neutrophilic and lymphocytic infiltrate. Epicutaneous patch testing may also support the diagnosis by causing a localized pustular reaction 48-96 hours after the offending drug is applied. The condition usually resolves by 15 days after the causative drug is withdrawn but oral corticosteroid therapy may be necessary in some individuals. The mortality rate is up to 5% and mostly occurs in the elderly who have significant comorbidities.

4. Stevens-Johnson Syndrome/Toxic Epidermal Necrolysis

4.1. History and nosology

SJS and TEN were once considered as variants of erythema multiforme (EM), a condition first described by Ferdinand von Hebra in 1860 [1] as a mild and relapsing eruption of target lesions affecting the acral regions. Mucosal involvement occurs in up to 70% of cases of EM. In 1922, two American paediatricians, Albert Stevens and Frank Johnson, described two cases of fever, stomatitis, purulent conjunctivitis, and a generalized eruption of purple papules in boys aged 7 and 8 years, respectively [2]. Both cases were distinguished from EM by the prolonged high fever, and the generalized distribution and heavy terminal crusting of the skin lesions. Bernard Thomas proposed two categories of EM in 1950: erythema multiforme minor, as described by von Hebra, and erythema multiforme major, a severe form that encompassed SJS [3]. Alan Lyell, a Scottish dermatologist, termed the condition toxic epidermal necrolysis (TEN) after reporting four cases of an acute life threatening mucocutaneous disorder characterized by diffuse erythema followed by extensive epidermal detachment manifesting as blistering and sloughing of the skin [4]. Although SJS and TEN were initially considered distinct entities, it was later proposed that they form a continuum along the same disease process and differ mainly in the extent of involvement [5],[6]. It was also proposed that EM major and SJS are distinct conditions, with EM major characterised by acral target-like lesion typical of EM minor but with mucosal involvement. SJS was applied to cases of mucous membrane involvement and a more extensive eruption of atypical targetoid lesions, blisters or sloughing of the skin [7]. The distinction between EM and SJS are consistent with observations regarding differences in etiology, demography and histopathology and not just confined to variations in the severity of disease. Most cases of EM are related to infection especially those with recurrent disease, which is related to herpes simplex virus (HSV) infection [8]-[10] in contrast to SJS which usually is an idiosyncratic reaction to drugs [11]. EM typically affects young adults in their 20s and 30s although approximately 20% of cases involve children [12],[13] whereas SJS/TEN occurs at any age [11]. Histopathology in EM in contrast to SJS/TEN consists of a denser infiltrate of lymphocytes and less apoptosis of keratinocytes [14].

In 1993, a classification scheme was proposed that is widely but not universally adopted that arbitrarily defines SJS and TEN according to the extent of epidermal detachment [7]. In SJS, epidermal loss affects less than 10% of the total body surface area (TBSA) whereas TEN involves greater than 30% of the TBSA. Epidermal detachment between 10 and 30% of the TBSA is classified as SJS/TEN overlap.

4.2. Epidemiology

The epidemiology of SJS/TEN and other severe cutaneous adverse reactions (SCARs) has been more accurately determined in recent years due to registries that have been established mainly across Europe comprising cases that are reviewed by expert committees and based on predefined and validated criteria. A population-based registry was commenced in Germany in 1990 to collect all hospitalised cases of SJS, TEN and EM major [15]. An international case-control study was conducted between 1989 and 1995 in France, Germany, Italy and Portugal

(SCAR study) focusing on cases of SJS/TEN requiring hospitalisation [16],[17]. A European case-control surveillance study of SCARs (EuroSCAR study) was conducted between 1997 and 2001 in Austria, France, Germany, Israel, Italy, and the Netherlands investigating both SJS/TEN [11] and AGEP [18] that resulted in admission to hospital. In 2003, the European registry on SCARs (RegiSCAR) was commenced collecting biological samples across the same countries that participated in the EuroSCAR study. This network, which is focused on SJS/TEN and AGEP, has spawned numerous studies on epidemiology, pharmacogenetics and histopathology and includes community cases that requiring hospitalisation as well as cases that developed during hospital admissions. These registries not only provide valuable information on the epidemiology of SCAR but they have enabled close scrutiny of the availability and prescription of high-risk drugs. For example, the SCAR study resulted in the withdrawal of chlormezanone from the market and restricted indications for cotrimoxazole and phenobarbitol [17].

The incidence of SJS/TEN is 1-2 cases/million inhabitants/year [15]. The EuroSCAR study published in 2008 comprised 379 cases that included 134 cases of SJS, 136 cases of SJS/TEN overlap, and 109 cases TEN spanning a geographical area encompassing over a 100 million inhabitants. The median age of cases was found to be 50 years (range 1-95 years), and a female preponderance (62% of cases) was noted [11].

4.3. Etiology

4.3.1. Drugs

Drugs are nearly always the cause of SJS/TEN. Over 220 medications have been implicated but only relatively a few are responsible for the majority of cases. The EuroSCAR study comprised 379 cases of SJS/TEN and 1505 age-matched controls, who were patients admitted to hospital for other acute illnesses [11]. Univariate relative risk (uRR) and multivariate relative risk (mRR) were calculated for each drug suspected of causing SJS/TEN. The drugs found to confer the highest risk were cotrimoxazole (uRR 102), other anti-bacterial sulphonamides (uRR 53), carbamazepine (mRR 72), nevirapine (uRR >22), allopurinol (mRR 18), phenytoin (mRR 17), oxicam-NSAIDs (mRR 16), lamotrigine (uRR >14), and sertraline (mRR 11). Drugs that were found to have a significant but lower risk included acetic acid-NSAIDs, macrolides, quinolones, cephalosporins, tetracyclines and aminopenicillins. SJS/TEN typically occurs with drugs that are taken on a long-term basis. The median latency between the onset of medication use and the occurrence of SJS/TEN in the EuroSCAR study was found to be less than 4 weeks (range 1-8 weeks): carbamazepine 15 days, phenobarbitol 17 days, allopurinol 20 days, phenytoin 24 days. Pantoprazole and tramadol were associated with high uRRs, 18 and 20, respectively, but the frequent co-medication with highly suspected drugs and the timing of the onset of SJS/TEN were not suggestive of a true risk. Commonly used medications not associated with a risk of SJS/TEN included beta-blockers, ACE-inhibitors, calcium channel blockers, thiazide diuretics, furosemide, propionic acid-NSAIDs, sulphonylureas, and insulin. Interestingly, valproic acid was not shown to have a significant risk, which is in contrast to previous observations [17],[19]. The most likely explanation is that valproic acid was frequently coadministered with high-risk drugs.

A pooled analysis of the SCAR and EuroSCAR data was performed for children under 15 years of age and showed that anti-bacterial sulphonamides, phenobarbitol, lamotrigine and carbamazepine were strongly associated with SJS/TEN in this paediatric population [20].

4.3.2. Other causes

Infection with *Mycoplasma pneumoniae* is a known cause of SJS especially in the paediatric population and a few cases of TEN have been reported to complicate infection with this agent [13],[21]. However, the EuroSCAR study, failed to show that infection is a risk factor on its own although there is a suggestion that it may modestly increase the risk of SJS/TEN from medication. SJS/TEN has been reported in association with vaccinations [22] and exposure to industrial chemicals and fumigants [23].

4.4. Clinical presentation

SJS/TEN is characterized, as per the original descriptions, by fever, blistering skin eruption and severe mucositis [2],[4]. The skin lesions initially appear as atypical target–like or targetoid lesions, which are erythematous macules that contain a central purpuric blister (Fig. 1). Lesions

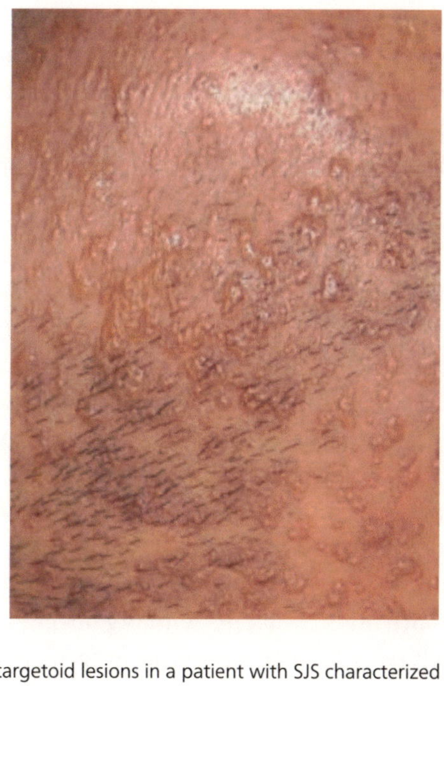

Figure 1. Atypical target-like or targetoid lesions in a patient with SJS characterized by an erythematous macule with a central blister.

are symmetrically distributed often starting on the face and thorax before spreading to other areas (Fig. 2). The scalp is typically spared. Blisters result from epidermal detachment and they are easily breached resulting in dark red oozing erosions. Lesions exhibit Nikolsky's sign, which is epidermal separation induced by gentle lateral pressure applied to the skin surface. The skin then sloughs rapidly over several days as a result of separation of large sheets of the epidermis from the dermis. Fulminant cases of TEN have been reported were total loss of the epidermis occurs within 24 hours [24]. New lesions may continue to erupt for up to 4 weeks. However, the growth of a new epithelium occurs after several days and individual lesions are completely re-epithelialized after a mean of 3 weeks. Cicatrization of the mucous membranes may take longer to complete.

At least two mucosal surfaces are involved in 90% of cases of SJS/TEN [25]. Oropharyngeal involvement causes severe pain and odynophagia as a result of erosion and crusting (Fig. 3). Ocular regions may show a purulent conjunctivitis, pseudomembrane formation and corneal ulceration as a result of sloughing of conjunctival and corneal epithelia (Fig. 4). Urethritis may result in dysuria and even urinary retention. Sloughing of the tracheal and bronchial epithelium occurs in up to 30% of cases and may result in hypoxia, bronchial hypersecretion, pulmonary edema and bronchiolitis obliterans and the need for mechanical ventilation [26], [27]. The gastrointestinal tract can also be involved resulting in per rectal bleeding [28].

The mortality of SJS is generally below 10% whereas 30-50% of TEN patients die in the acute phase of the illness mostly as a result of skin failure. Infection and sepsis with multiorgan failure is the most common of death. The causative organisms are usually *Staphylococcus aureus* and *Pseudomonas aeruginosa* [29]. Fluid and electrolyte imbalances occur as a result of increased transepidermal water loss and impaired intake of nutrition due to odynophagia from stomatitis. Less common fatal complications include adult respiratory distress syndrome, pulmonary embolism and gastrointestinal haemorrhage [30],[31]. Mortality is accurately predicted by the SCORTEN scale (Table 1) and should be computed within 24 hours and 3 days following admission [32]-[34].

Chronic complications occur frequently following the acute phase of SJS/TEN. The most serious sequelae relate to the eye. The chronic ocular consequences are that of a cicatrization of the conjunctiva and symblepharon formation, severe dry eye, trichiasis, eyelid margin keratinization, and limbal stem cell deficiency, all of which combine to cause corneal ulceration and scarring and loss of vision (Fig. 5) [35],[36]. Patients may also experience chronic photophobia and eye pain [37]. Skin sequelae include scarring, pigmentation abnormalities, and shedding of hair and nails [38]. Vulvovaginal involvement can result in stenosis [39]. Vulvar adenosis can occur in young women several years after resolution of the acute episode and can present with tender, erosive, haemorrhagic lesions [40]. Phimosis can occur in men [41]. Bronchopulmonary complications confer a poor prognosis and include chronic bronchitis, bronchiolitis obliterans, bronchiolitis obliterans with organizing pneumonia, bronchiectasis [42],[43] Oesophageal stricture and webbing has also been described and can result in dysphagia [44].

http://dx.doi.org/10.5772/54820

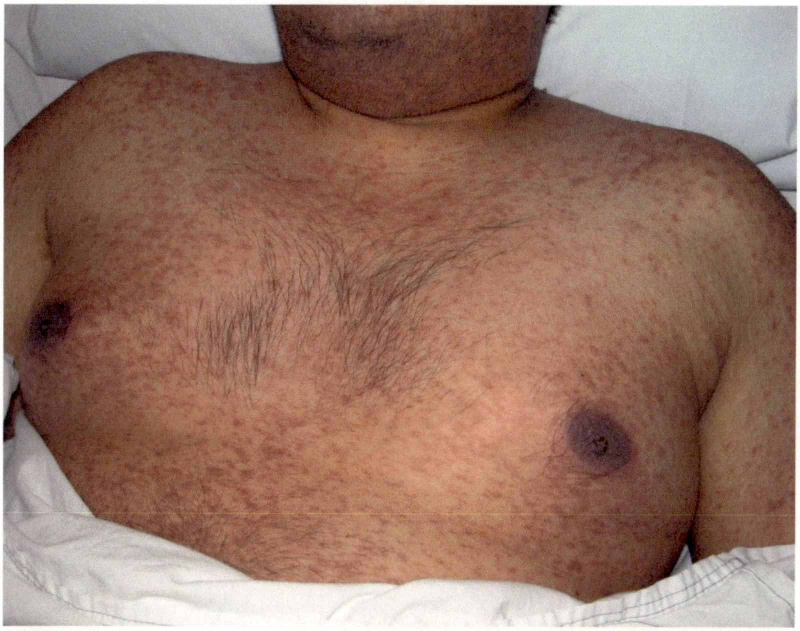

(a)

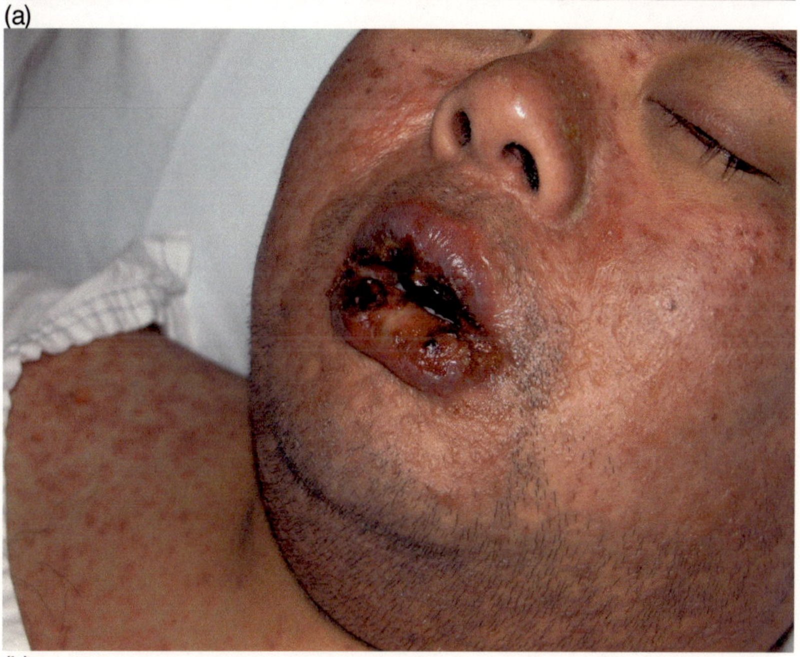

(b)

Figure 2. Symmetrical distribution of targetoid lesions in a patient with SJS, which typically first appear on the face and thorax before spreading to other areas.

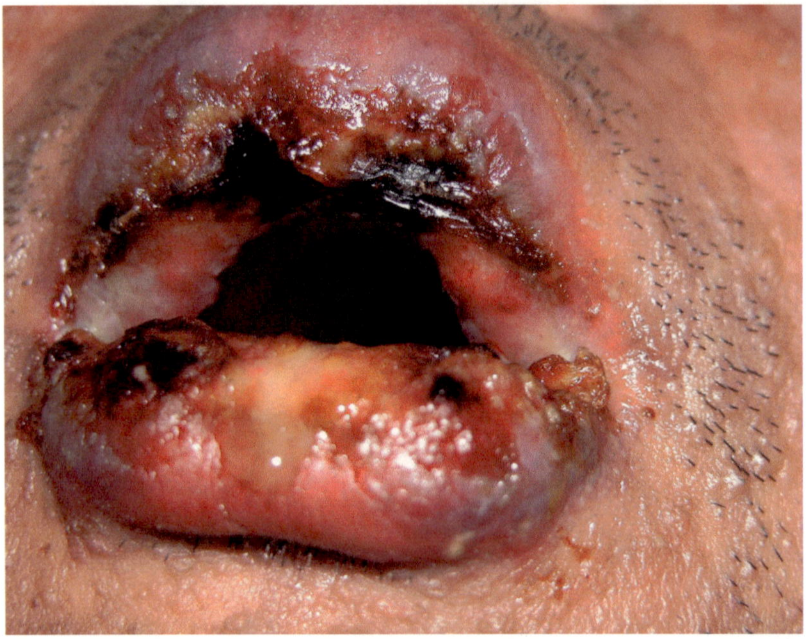

Figure 3. Oral mucositis in a patient with SJS depicted as sloughing, necrosis and crusting of the inner labial surfaces.

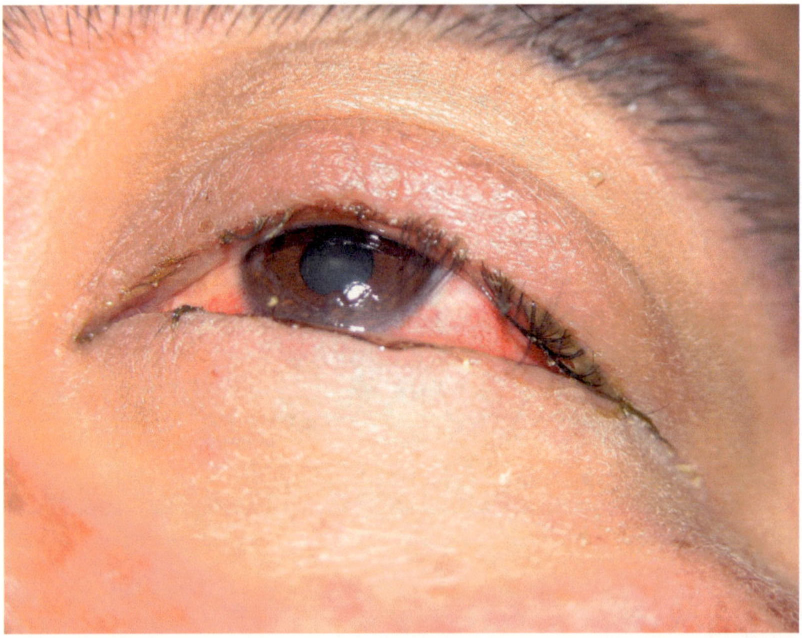

Figure 4. Purulent conjunctivitis in a patient with SJS accompanied by pseudomembrane formation, which results from sloughing of conjunctival and corneal surfaces.

Severe Cutaneous Adverse Reactions	**Severe Cutaneous Adverse Reactions**
Age >40 years	1
Presence of malignancy	1
Heart rate >120/min	1
TBSA involved >10%	1
Serum urea > 10 mmol/L (28 mg/dL)	1
Serum glucose >14 mmol/L (252 mg/dL)	1
Serum bicarbonate <20 mmol/L (20 mEq/L)	1
SCORTEN	Mortality (%)
0-1	3.2
2	12.1
3	35.3
4	58.3
≥5	90

Table 1. SCORTEN

4.5. Pathogenesis

SJS/TEN results from the T- and NK-cell mediated extensive apoptosis of keratinocytes. The pharmaco-immune (p-i) concept, the mechanism by which the drug binds directly with the T cell receptor (TCR) causing activation of proapoptotic pathways. Granulysin is the major mediator of apoptosis in SJS/TEN. Apoptosis is also mediated through involved Fas-FasL interaction, and the release of granzyme and perforin.

4.5.1. The pharmaco-immune (p-i) concept

It is generally accepted that in SJS/TEN, the parent drug binds directly and non-covalently to the MHC and the TCR of primed effector and memory T cells [45]. Naïve T cells are not sufficiently stimulated by a p-i drug and additional signals are required [46]. T cells may be primed by infection or autoimmune disease resulting in high cytokine levels such as IL-2 and IFN-γ resulting in increased expression of MHC and costimulatory molecules. This may provide an explanation for the increased incidence of drug hypersensitivity in inflammatory and infectious diseases. The drug may also bind to toll-like receptors resulting in the expression of costimulatory molecules by dendritic cells. For drugs such as cotrimoxazole, lamotrigine, and carbamazepine, the p-i concept may not be the sole mechanism involved; metabolites may also play a role through haptenization [47].

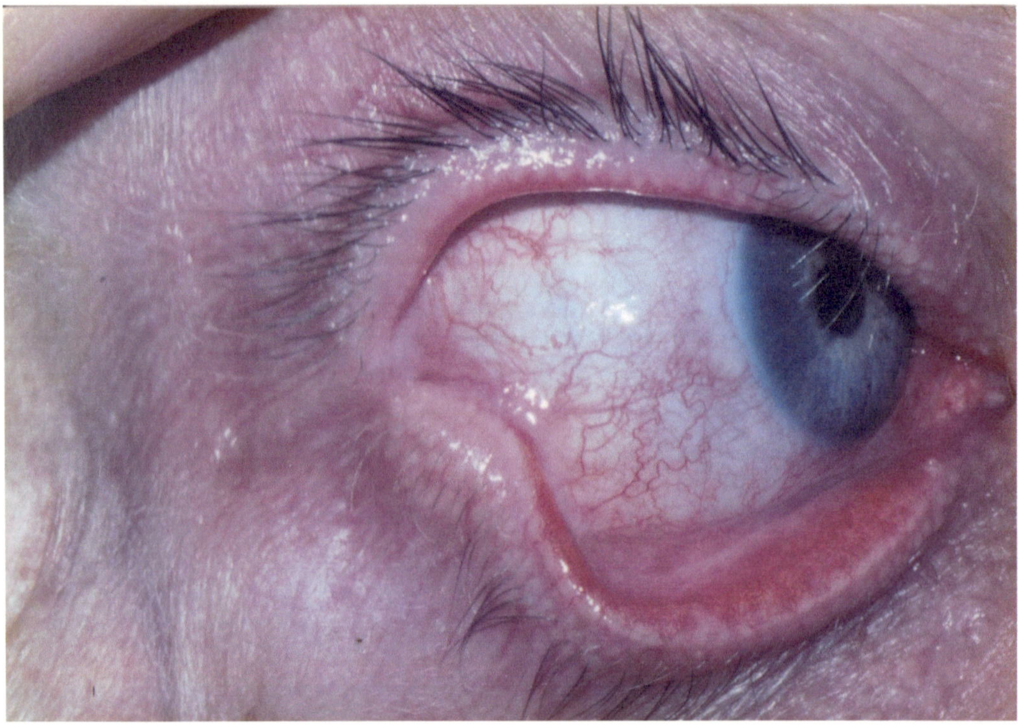

Figure 5. Cicatrization of the bulbar and palpebral conjunctival surfaces with resultant symblepharon formation, shortening of the fornix, and distichiasis.

4.5.2. Granulysin

A recent study by Chung et al using global gene expression profiling showed that granulysin RNA was the most significant cytotoxic molecule expressed in blister cells from patients with SJS/TEN. Granulysin protein concentrations were 2-4 times higher than perforin, granzyme B, and FasL and depleting granulysin reduced cytotoxicity [48]. Granulysin is a cationic cytolytic protein produced by CTL, NK and NKT cells [49]. The 15-kDa-precursor form, found in blister fluid, induced skin necrosis when injected into mice and exhibited significant cytotoxicity in vitro. This contrasted with the minimal cytotoxicity induced by perforin, granzyme B, and FasL [48]. Granulysin is also a proinflammatory molecule that causes an increase in the expression of chemokines (RANTES/CCL5, MCP-1, MCP-3, MIP-1α/CCL3) and cytokines (IL-1, IL-6, IFN-α) resulting in the recruitment of T cells, monocytes and other inflammatory cells [50].

4.5.3. Fas-FasL, perforin/ granzyme and TNF pathways

Viard et al, showed that the binding of FasL to Fas expressed on the surface of keratinocytes resulted in their apoptosis [51]. The cytoplasmic death domain of Fas undergoes conformational changes and trimerization upon recognition of FasL. This results in the recruitment of the Fas-associated death domain (FADD), which binds to procaspase 8 resulting in triggering

http://dx.doi.org/10.5772/54820

of the caspase cascade and apoptosis. The source of the FasL is unclear. Viard et al showed that the FasL was is present on the surface of keratinocytes and in the serum of patients with TEN but not on the surface of keratinocytes or in the serum of patients with maculopapular exanthems and normal controls [51]. A further study demonstrated that FasL was not constitutively expressed on the surface of keratinocytes but are transported to the cell membrane after damage to the keratinocyte [52]. Abe et al, however, found that the source of FasL was PBMCs and not keratinocytes [53].

Nassif et al showed that mononuclear cells from blister fluid induce cytotoxicity via perforin and granzyme B [54]. This cytotoxicity was blocked by inhibiting perforin/granzyme but not by inhibiting Fas. Perforin and granzyme are proteins stored in the granules of CTLs. Upon recognition of a target cell, the CTL releases perforin, which create 16-nm channels in the target cell membrane. Granzyme B, a protease passes through these channels to activate the caspase cascade. The loss of T regulatory cell function in the acute stage of SJS/TEN may further contribute to the epidermal damage caused by effector T cells [55].

Posadas et al, showed that both Fas-FasL and perforin/granzyme pathways may be involved in SJS/TEN. They found a direct correlation between disease severity and levels of perforin and granzyme B in patients with maculopapular exanthems, SJS and TEN. FasL was detected in the PBMCs and blister fluid of patients in SJS and TEN but not in those in maculopapular exanthema, suggesting that Fas-FasL is involved in more severe reactions [56].

Nassif et al, also showed a potential role for cytokines in the pathogenesis of SJS/TEN. He found elevated levels of IFN-γ, soluble TNF, IL-10, soluble FasL in the blister fluid of TEN patients. Although they disputed the central role of FasL, they hypothesised that drug specific CTLs secrete IFN-γ, which activates keratinocytes to produce TNF, a cytokine that upregulated MHC class I molecules. This increases exposure of keratinocytes to CTL resulting in perforin/granzyme-mediated apoptosis. IL-10 serves to downregulate the inflammatory reaction [57].

More recently, TRAIL (TNF related apoptosis inducing ligand) and TWEAK (TNF-like weak inducer of apoptosis) were shown to be present in blister fluid from TEN patients [36]. They are released by CD1a and CD14 cells and initiate apoptosis of keratinocytes in a MHC-class I-independent manner.

4.6. Risk factors for SJS/TEN

4.6.1. Genetic susceptibility

It was observed in the 1990s that the most commonly offending drugs varied among different ethnic populations. In Western countries, the most commonly implicated agents of SJS/TEN were NSAIDs and sulphonamides [17]. In contrast, carbamazepine was found to be the leading cause of SJS/TEN in Southeast Asian countries, including India, Malaysia, Singapore, Taiwan and Hong Kong [58]. Interestingly, carbamazepine in Western countries causes more cases of DIHS than SJS/TEN. Allopurinol is also a frequent case of SJS/TEN and DIHS but does not appear to have a racial bias [59].

The most striking genetic association was detected in a cohort of Han Chinese in Taiwan, where the *HLA-B*1502* allele was found in 100% of the 44 patients with carbamazepine-induced SJS/TEN and only 3% of the carbamazepine-tolerant individuals; OR 2504 [126–49522] [60]. These findings were replicated in an extended cohort of subjects of Chinese descent originating from separated geographic areas of China, Taiwan, and the United States [61]. This association with carbamazepine-induced SJS/TEN, however, was not found in individuals with European [62] and Japanese ancestries [63], respectively, and therefore the allele appears relevant in the context of ethnicity. In a recent study comprising 12 patients of Northern European ancestry with carbamazepine-induced SJS/TEN, 5 (42%) carried the *HLA-A*3101* allele, as compared with 10 (4%) of the 257 control subjects; OR 25.93 [4.93-116.18] [64]. The results of this study are yet to be replicated in other cohorts of subjects with Northern European ancestry. In a Japanese study, The *HLA-A*3101* allele was found in 5/6 (83.3%) carbamazepine-induced SJS/TEN compared to 47/376 (12.5%) carbamazepine-tolerant patients; OR 33.9 [3.9-295.6]. Larger patient sample sizes are required to confirm this association in the Japanese where the allele frequency is 9% [65]. Interestingly the *HLA-A*3101* allele was shown to be associated with maculopapular exanthem (OR 17.5 [4.6-66.5]) but not SJS/TEN in a Han Chinese population [66].

A study comprising a Han Chinese cohort in Taiwan demonstrated the presence of the *HLA-B*5801* allele in all 51 patients with allopurinol-induced SCAR (21 with TEN, 30 with DIHS) compared with only 15% (20/135) in allopurinol-tolerant subjects; OR 580.3 [34.4-9780.9] [67].

The role of these HLA alleles in the pathogenesis of SCAR is unclear. Certain HLA alleles may bind to particular drugs more robustly than other alleles. Furthermore, the binding of the drug in SJS/TEN is MHC class I restricted, which is consistent with the prominent role of CD8 cells in the pathogenesis of the disease. If an allele has a functional effect that may play a role in the pathogenesis of disease, this association will be consistently observed across different populations. The differences observed between the Chinese and European studies may be partly explained by the fact that pharmacogenetic studies are likely to yield positive results when conducted in a population with a high frequency of such an allele [69]. The risk of disease from a genetic polymorphism is influenced by its prevalence. The *HLA-B*1502* allele frequency is 4.8 to 12.8% in Southeast Asians compared to 0-0.1% observed in Northern Europeans [58]. For instance, *HLA-B*1502* is of low prevalence in Caucasians and hence, if it is a true susceptibility allele, a very large sample size is required in this population to detect a significant odds ratio of sufficient power. In contrast, the allele frequency of *HLA-A*3101* is 2-5% in Northern Europeans [70] and the sample size required to demonstrate an association in a sufficiently powered study is less than that for the *HLA-B*1502* allele. The *HLA-B*5801* allele, in contrast to *HLA-B*1502* is more evenly distributed among different racial groups [59] and hence, associations, albeit weaker, have been demonstrated in other ethnic groups such as the Southern Japanese [63] and in whites (OR 80 [34-157]) [68].

Another explanation is that *HLA-B*1502*, is a marker of a true disease contributing allele through strong linkage disequilibrium, which varies between populations. In other words, the same high-risk allele may have a different pattern of association with marker alleles and therefore *HLA-B*1502* is in strong linkage disequilibrium in the Han Chinese population, but

http://dx.doi.org/10.5772/54820

not in a European population. It is also plausible is that SJS/TEN is a polygenic disorder, with many susceptibility and protective alleles in genes involved in the pathogenesis of the disease. Polymorphisms in the proapoptotic gene *Fas-L* [71], the toll-like receptor 3 gene [72], and in the IL-4 receptor/IL-13 signalling pathway [73] have all been recently described in a Japanese study. Such alleles may also vary in different populations.

The FDA and Health Canada have issued warnings for carbamazepine stating that persons with ancestry in genetically at-risk populations should be screened for the presence of *HLA-B*1502* prior to initiating treatment [74]. Genetic screening for *HLA-B*1502* in a high risk population such as the Han Chinese has a 100% sensitivity and 97% specificity and its presence confers a 7.7% positive predictive value for carbamazepine-induced SJS/TEN whereas its absence has a 100% negative predictive value [58]. The odds ratio in test-positive Chinese patients to test-negative patients of having carbamazepine-induced SJS/TEN is >3200. Although 3% of patients who are test-positive may never develop the disease, the serious and life-threatening consequences of developing SJS/TEN and the availability of alternative drugs, justifies its exclusion from these individuals. The lack of prevalence of *HLA-B*1502* in non-Asian populations may limit its cost effectiveness as a screening tool in these populations and cannot be currently recommended. A recent study demonstrated the benefit of genetic screening; in a Taiwanese population, screening for the *HLA-B*1502* allele resulted in no cases of SJS/TEN in 4501 patients who were negative for the allele [75]. The authors concluded that this would have prevented 10 cases of SJS/TEN. Despite the FDA recommendations, screening is not routinely performed partly because of the lack of availability of cost effective and rapid methods of detection [76]. Susceptibility alleles can be identified by high resolution sequence based HLA typing after a 20 ml sample of blood is collected in an ADC tube. However, this highly specialized and relatively expensive diagnostic technique is limited to a small number of laboratories that focus on transplantation medicine and may be limited by longer turn-around times of up to 3-4 weeks. Many laboratories have now developed high resolution genetic testing using a sequence-specific primer assay method for the detection of this allele from samples collected in either 7-10 ml of whole blood (EDTA tube) or buccal swabs (provided by the testing laboratory). The assay can be performed within 3-4 hours. Such a strategy is not novel and has been very successful in virtually abolishing the incidence of *HLA-B*5701*-associated abacavir hypersensitivity in HIV-infected patients [77]. Multiplexed PCRs can be utilized to assess multiple alleles.

It is important to note that the *HLA-B*1502* allele does not predispose to carbamazepine-induced DIHS, maculopapular eruptions or other adverse reactions and continued vigilance for the symptoms of SCAR needs to be maintained if treatment is commenced [61].

Currently, there is no recommendation for genetic screening prior to the commencement of allopurinol therapy. Although such a strategy is plausible, studies are required to determine the benefits of screening for the *HLA*5801* allele in at risk populations.

4.6.2. Diseases

The EuroSCAR study showed that HIV infection conferred the highest risk of SJS/TEN; multivariate relative risk (mvRR) 12 [2.4-59]. Other disease associations included collagen vascular disease mvRR 2.2 [0.9-5.0], recent malignancy mvRR 2.7 [1.3-5.7], recent radiotherapy mvRR 2.1 [0.5-9.0], or acute infection in the past 4 weeks [1.2-2.3] [11].

4.6.3. Pharmacokinetics

The EuroSCAR study revealed an increased risk of SJS/TEN at higher doses of allopurinol; adjusted odds ratio (OR) 36 [17-76] for doses ≥200 mg daily compared with an adjusted OR 3.0 [1.1-8.4] for doses <200 mg daily [78]. This study also revealed that the risk was mostly confined to short-term use (≤8 weeks, unadjusted OR 261 [36-∞]). Allopurinol should be commenced at a dose of 100 mg daily and increased by 100 mg increments until the desired serum uric acid level is attained. Previous reports have shown that allopurinol is commenced at inappropriate doses [79] and that higher doses are associated with an increased incidence of acute events [80]. It is likely that the rapid accumulation of the chemically reactive metabolite oxypurinol when higher doses of allopurinol are commenced increases the risk of SJS/TEN [81],[82]. This drug accumulation hypothesis is further supported by the 4.7 fold increased incidence of allopurinol-induced SCAR in renal insufficiency [83]. The established indications for allopurinol are treatment of hyperuricemia associated with chronic gout, acute uric acid nephropathy, recurrent uric acid stone formation, enzyme disorders of purine metabolism, and in the management of tumour lysis. Allopurinol is not indicated in the majority of patients with asymptomatic hyperuricemia [84]. However, allopurinol is inappropriately prescribed in up to 86% of cases [85]-[87]. A comparison of allopurinol exposure between the SCAR (1989-1993) and EuroSCAR (1997-2001) studies showed a 2-3 fold increase in exposure for both patients and control subjects, which may be attributed to the increased prescribing of the drug for the treatment of asymptomatic hyperuricemia. The authors of the EuroSCAR study postulate that up to 48 of the 56 cases of allopurinol-induced SJS/TEN could have been prevented if the treatment guidelines for prescribing allopurinol were followed.

Lamotrigine when commenced at high doses can also overwhelm the detoxifying capacity resulting in an increased risk of SJS/TEN and DIHS [88]. The incidence has reduced significantly as a result of the now conventional practice of gradually titrating the dose [89]. Coadministration of certain drugs can predispose to SCAR by competition for the same enzyme-binding site. Reactions to lamotrigine are more common when given in combination with valproic acid as the addition of valproic acid inhibits the clearance of lamotrigine by competing for glucoronic acid conjugation [90].

The role of slow acetylation phenotypes of N-acetyltransferase was thought to confer susceptibility of sulphonamide-induced SJS/TEN in two small studies [91],[92] but this needs confirmation in larger studies.

4.7. Diagnosis

A presumptive diagnosis of SJS/TEN is made clinically and is confirmed with a skin biopsy (Figs. 6 & 7). Early lesions demonstrate vacuolar alteration and scattered necrotic keratinocytes in the epidermal layers at the level of the stratum spinosum and the basal cell layer. Later, full thickness epidermal necrosis is evident, which eventuates in the formation of subepidermal bullae [93]. The mononuclear predominantly T cell dermal infiltrate is generally sparse but dense infiltrates can also be present. Quinn et al, has shown an extensive infiltrate was associated with a 71% mortality rate, a moderate infiltrate with a 53% mortality, and a sparse infiltrate with a 27% mortality, respectively [94]. A fresh sample for direct immunofluoresence (DIF) reveals an absence of immunoglobulin and complement deposition. The cornified layer remains intact. Immunohistochemistry usually reveals a predominance of CD8 cells in the epidermis and CD4 cells in the dermis. A fresh sample for direct immunofluoresence (DIF) reveals an absence of immunoglobulin and complement deposition.

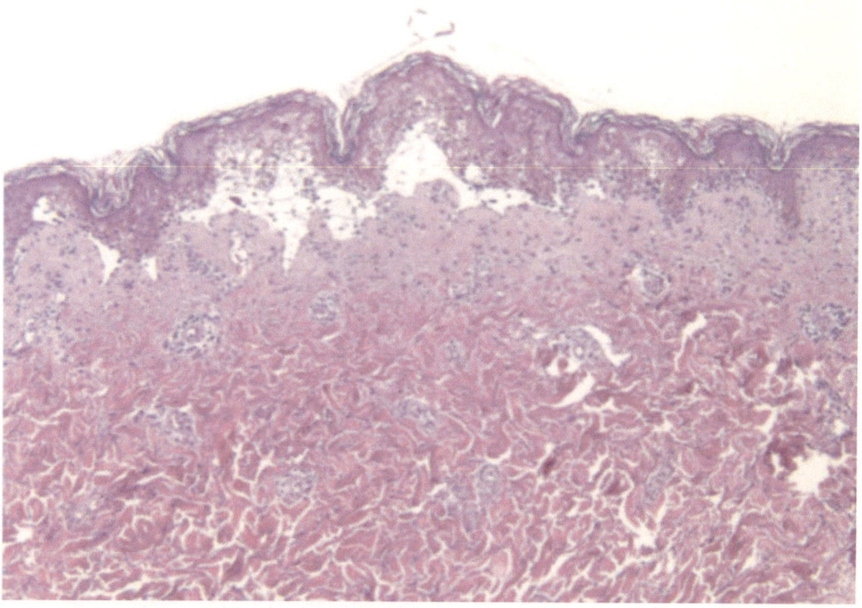

Figure 6. Low power view of a skin biopsy from a patient with SJS demonstrates separation of the epidermis from the dermis at the level of the stratum spinosum and basal cell layer resulting in the formation of subepidermal bullae (Hematoxylin-eosin, original magnification x40).

Cultures on blood, wounds and mucosal lesions should be performed to evaluate for superinfection. Serology may be performed for *Mycoplasma pneumoniae* if indicated.

A recent pilot study showed that serum granulysin levels may be raised early in the course of disease but rapidly wanes with progression of disease [95]. Further studies are required to determine whether this assay will prove to be a useful early diagnostic test for SJS/TEN.

4.8. Allergy testing

Skin tests and oral challenges are contraindicated in SJS/TEN because of the risk of inducing a recurrence of disease. Patch testing has not been investigated extensively. The biggest cohort comprised 22 patients and showed a poor sensitivity of only 9% [96]. Lymphocyte transformation tests (LTTs) assesses the proliferation of the patient's peripheral blood T cells cultured

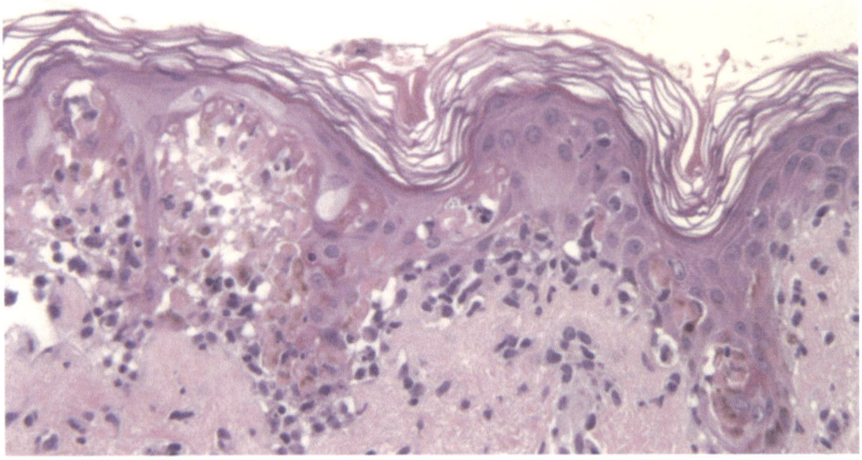

Figure 7. High power view of a skin biopsy from a patient with SJS shows necrosis of keratinocytes, and vacuolar degeneration of the basal cell layer. A sparse lymphocytic infiltrate is present at the dermoepidermal junction and displays satellitosis or clustering around dying basal cells (Hematoxylin-eosin, original magnification x200).

in the presence of a suspected drug for 6 days by measuring the incorporation of ^{3}H-thymidine during DNA synthesis. The result is expressed as a stimulation index, which is the ratio of cell proliferation with antigen and without antigen. The sensitivity of LTTs in SJS/TEN is greatly improved if the test is performed within 1 week of the onset of disease but becomes negative by 6 weeks [97]. This may be attributed to loss of regulatory T cell function in the acute phase, which is then restored upon recovery [55]. Recently, a new cytotoxicity assay combining the measurement of expression of the degranulation marker, CD107a, using flow cytometry and the release of the serine protease, granzyme B by Elispot after incubating the patient's peripheral blood mononuclear cells with the suspected drug for 3 days [98]. The test has very good specificity with all of the 16 controls having a negative test and good sensitivity with 10 of the 12 patients having a positive result. One role of these in vitro tests is to determine the culprit drug when more than one drug is suspected.

4.9. Differential Diagnosis

SJS/TEN is differentiated from other conditions on the basis of the acute onset of disease, the presence of targetoid and vesiculobullous lesions, sloughing of the epidermis, severe mucosal involvement, the histologic finding of full thickness epidermal necrosis, and a negative DIF. In EM major, erosive mucous membrane involvement is present but in contrast to SJS, the patient has typical target lesions mainly affecting the extremities and it is often induced by acute or recurrent HSV infection. The clinical manifestations of drug-induced maculopapular exanthems (MPE) are variable and often polymorphic and lesions may have a target-like appearance. Fever may be present but mucosal involvement is absent. The histopathology typically shows an interface dermatitis with hydropic degeneration of the basal cell layer [99]. Some exanthems may progress to more severe reactions such as SJS/TEN or DIHS. Generalized bullous fixed drug eruption (GBFDE) features large brownish violaceous patches upon which flaccid blisters arise. These blisters affect only a small percentage of the TBSA. Mucosal involvement is rare and fever is absent. Most patients report a history of a similar local reaction or fixed drug eruption [100].

Staphylococcal scalded skin syndrome (SSSS) usually affects children under the age of 5 years and patients present with fever, erythema and painful skin, followed by blistering, which is typically accentuated in areas of friction and around orifices [101]. SSSS is caused by the systemic distribution of epidermolytic toxins produced by certain strains of Staphylococci. These toxins cause separation at the level of the stratum granulosum, the upper layer of the epidermis, resulting in very superficial detachment of the skin and blistering[102]. Mucous membrane involvement is rare. The condition usually but not always follows local or systemic staphylococcal infection [103]. Adults are less susceptible as improved renal function allows for better clearance of the toxins. However SSSS has been described in adults who are immunosuppressed or in renal failure [101]. Toxic shock syndrome (TSS) is caused by elaboration of toxins produced by *Staphylococcus aureus* and *Streptococcus pyogenes* that act as superantigens, which bind to the variable regions of β chains of antigen receptors on subsets of T cells and cross-link them to the MHC molecules of antigen-presenting cells [104]. This results in activation of large numbers of T cells (5-30%) and the massive release of cytokines including IL-2, TNF, lymphotoxin and IL-1β. TSS is characterised by fever, diffuse red macular rash, hypotension and involvement of ≥3 organs: renal failure, hepatitis, thrombocytopenia, encephalopathy, mucous membrane hyperemia, gastrointestinal involvement with vomiting and diarhhoea. Desquamation occurs after 1-2 weeks and predominantly affects the palms and soles. Approximately 50% of cases are menstrually related due to the prolonged application of absorbent tampons. Notably, 50% of cases of TSS are not associated with menstruation. Non-menstrual cases of TSS usually complicate the use of barrier contraceptives, surgical and postpartum wound infections, burns, cutaneous lesions, osteomyelitis, and arthritis. Although most cases of TSS occur in women, about 25% of non-menstrual cases occur in men.

Autoimmune bullous diseases need to be considered in the differential diagnosis of SJS/TEN. These conditions, in contrast to SJS/TEN, usually have a chronic course and are characterized by acantholysis on histopathology and immunoglobulin deposition on DIF. Drug-induced linear IgA bullous dermatosis can produce an acute extensive eruption of target-like lesions, pruritic urticarial plaques and tense bullae on the trunk and limbs [105]. Vancomycin is the most commonly implicated drug. In contrast to SJS, mucosal lesions are rare and DIF shows linear deposition of IgA at the basement membrane zone. Paraneoplastic pemphigus (PNP) is a chronic disease characterized by severe and intractable oral mucositis and a generalized polymorphous blistering eruption in association with an occult or overt malignancy, especially, lymphoma and Castleman's disease [106], [107]. Conjunctivitis is common and respiratory and gastrointestinal surfaces may be involved. DIF shows deposition of IgG and complement (C3) within the epidermal intercellular spaces and along the epidermal basement membrane. Drug-induced pemphigus is usually triggered by thiol drugs in genetically susceptible individuals [108]. These drugs, such as penicillamine, captopril and enalapril, directly interact with the epidermis and cause acantholysis and a superficial blistering eruption with crusts and erosions without mucosal involvement resembling pemphigus foliaceus (PF) [109]. However, in contrast to PF, which is mediated by antibodies against desmoglein-3, DIF may be negative in drug-induced pemphigus. Non-thiol drugs can cause disease indistinguishable from pemphigus vulgaris (PV). These cases of drug-triggered pemphigus, like PV are chronic with autoantibodies formed against desmoglein-3 [110]. Hence a flaccid blistering eruption with mucosal involvement occurs, and DIF shows IgG and C3 deposition in the epidermal intercellular spaces. Bullous pemphigoid (BP) is a chronic disease that is typified by a tense bullous eruption that primarily affects individuals in the fifth through seventh decades of life. Drugs, especially diuretics such as furosemide and spironolactone, can induce BP [111] and should be considered when the condition occurs in a young patient and the course is more abrupt [112]. Unlike in SJS/TEN, fever is absent, mucosal lesions are usually absent, and DIF reveals IgG and C3 linear deposition along the epidermal basement membrane [113].

Acute graft versus host disease (AGVHD) shares many of the same clinical, pathologic and immunologic features as SJS/TEN. Both conditions are mediated by cytotoxic T cells, which results in epidermal necrosis and keratinolysis [114],[115]. Furthermore, bone marrow transplantation (BMT) patients receive medications that can trigger SJS/TEN. AGVHD generally occurs 4 weeks after stem cell transplantation. Patients describe a sensation of skin pain and itching followed by a morbilliform rash that in severe cases becomes generalized with diffuse areas of epidermal necrosis [116]. Mucositis is usually present. AGVHD frequently begins acrally and spreads proximally in contrast to TEN, which begins on the trunk and spreads distally. Also, the early exanthem of AGVHD has a folliculocentric distribution [117].

AGEP is characterized by fever and as the disease progresses, widespread erosions mimicking SJS/TEN may be evident [118]. Mucous membrane involvement is unusual and if present is mild.

SJS/TEN, Stevens-Johnson syndrome/toxic epidermal necrolysis; EM, erythema multiforme; MPE, maculopapular exanthem; GBFDE, generalized bullous fixed drug eruption; SSSS, staphylococcal scalded skin syndrome; TSS, toxic shock syndrome; PNP, paraneoplastic pemphigus; AGVHD, acute graft versus host disease; AGEP, acute generalized exanthematous pustulosis

4.10. Treatment

4.10.1. Supportive care

Immediate discontinuation of the culprit drug is mandatory to reduce mortality [119]. As the management of TEN is similar to that of extensive burns, a transfer to a burns unit reduces morbidity and mortality. The largest trial showed a mortality rate of 29.8% after transfer to a burns unit compared to 51.4% ($p < .05$) after 7 days [120]. The unit has expertise in providing

http://dx.doi.org/10.5772/54820

Bullous disease	Fever	Mucositis	Rash	DIF	Onset	Other notable features
SJS/TEN	+	+	Erythroderma Targetoid lesions Vesicles, bullae Erosions, detachment	-	Acute	Starts on trunk, proximal upper limbs and face and then spreads
EM Major	+	+	Acral Target lesions	-	Acute	HSV-induced recurrences
Drug-induced MPE	+/-	-	Variable Pleomorphic	-	Acute	May progress to SJS or DIHS
GBFDE	-	-	Brown patches Large bullae	-	Acute	Antecedent local reaction Small % TBSA
SSSS	+	-	Erythroderma Skin tenderness Periorificial crusting	-	Acute	Children under 5 Adults with chronic renal failure and on immunosuppressive therapy
TSS	+	+	Diffuse red macular rash Desquamation of palms and soles	-	Acute	Hypotension Multiple organ failure
Drug-induced linear IgA dermatosis	-	-	Tense bullae	+	Acute	Vancomycin Pruritus
PNP	-	+	Polymorphous Bullae	+	Gradual	
Drug-induced pemphigus	-	-	Erosions Crusts	+	Gradual	Thiol drugs
Drug-triggered pemphigus	-	+	Mucosal erosions Flaccid bullae	+	Gradual	Non-thiol drugs
AGVHD	+	+	Morbilliform rash Bullae Erosions, detachment	-	Acute	Starts acrally and then spreads
AGEP	+	+/-	Small nonfollicular pustules Erythroderma	-	Acute	

Table 2. The differential diagnosis of SJS/TEN

analgesia, maintaining fluid and electrolyte balance and preventing and treating superinfection. It has been recently noted that in contrast to burns, TEN affects the epidermis and hence fluid and electrolyte requirements are less than for burns of the same extent [121]; initial administration of 2 ml/kg/%TBSA is usually sufficient [122]. Additional nutritional requirements result from loss of nitrogen and energy from the wound exudate, the hypermetabolic response of TEN and sepsis and the promotion of wound healing. However, these requirements may lower than in burns, with one study in the paediatric population suggesting that that patients with TENS require 22% fewer calories per day than patients with burns. A formula was subsequently developed: calorie requirement = baseline weight (kg) x 24.6 + wound size (%TBSA) x 4.1 + 940 [123]. Enteral or total parenteral nutrition should be considered in patients unable to ingest food. Nasogastric feeding should be cautiously initiated because of gastrointestinal involvement from TEN and the difficulties in placing a nasogastric tube in the presence of a oropharyngeal involvement [124]. Room temperature should be adjusted to 30-32ºC or heat-air body warmers should be used to prevent excessive caloric expenditure due to epidermal loss [25].

The optimal approach to wound management has not been determined and will therefore vary between specialty units. The contrasting measures of surgical debridement with whirlpool therapy to remove necrotic epidermis, and anti-shear wound care [125], in which detached skin is left in situ to act as a biological dressing [126], both have equivalent rates of re-epithelialization and survival. Non-adherent nanocrystalline-containing gauzes are being increasingly used because of their broad antimicrobial effects [127],[128]. This obviates the need for topical silver sulphadiazine because of the strong association between sulphonamides and SJS/TEN. There is also a trend in the use of biosynthetic skin substitutes in place of porcine xenograft and human allograft cadaveric skin because of reduced pain and improved mobilization in elderly patients [129].

Prophylactic antibiotics are not advised as they predispose to the emergence of resistant organisms [121]. Hence, repeated cultures of the skin, blood and other sites guide the need for antibiotic therapy. Sterile handling and reverse-isolation procedures are essential in the prevention of nosocomial infection [130].

Ophthalmologic consultation is mandatory in SJS/TEN and the combination of aggressive lubrication, topical antibiotics, topical corticosteroids, and lysis of adhesions with a glass rod is implemented immediately but has only a modest effect on the long term ocular complications. Recently, the application of amniotic membranes has proved effective in preserving visual acuity and an intact ocular surface [37]. The benefit may be derived from creating a physical barrier between inflamed and denuded mucosal surfaces that minimizes the formation of adhesions. The membrane may also have antiinflammatory and antifibrotic effects [131].

Other supportive measures include hygienic mouthwashes and topical oral anaesthetics, and monitoring for urinary retention.

4.10.2. Corticosteroids

The role of corticosteroids in the treatment of SJS/TEN is controversial. Corticosteroids given 48 hours or more prior to admission are associated with an increase incidence of infection, length of hospital admission, and mortality in children and adults [132]-[134]. A study in 1986 of 30 patients with TEN with an average TBSA involvement > 80% were equally divided into those receiving supportive care alone and those receiving dexamethasone at varying doses [135]. Although the incidence of sepsis was not significant different between the groups, the survival following onset of sepsis was less in the corticosteroid treated group. The use of corticosteroids doubled the rate of mortality (66% versus 33%). Corticosteroids do not prevent SJS/TEN from occurring and have no effect on arresting disease progression [136],[137]. A retrospective analysis of 281 patients from the EuroSCAR study found no benefit from corticosteroids or IVIg compared to supportive care alone.

The poor outcomes may have resulted from inadequate doses and the delay in the initiation of corticosteroid therapy. In a prospective study of 16 children with SJS in 1997, 10 received methylprednisolone (4 mg/kg/daily) within 3 days of the onset of rash whilst 6 received supportive care only; corticosteroids were associated with decreased length of fever and duration of skin eruption [138]. The use of pulsed IV corticosteroids has been shown in retrospective reviews to reduce mortality [139]-[141]. The initiation of IV methylprednisolone 500-1000 mg/daily for 3-4 days may also prevent ocular complications of cicatrization and preservation of visual acuity [142]. The benefits of early pulsed therapy with IV corticosteroids need to be further evaluated in randomized control trials.

The current level of evidence suggests that high dose corticosteroids may be beneficial if commenced early in the course of disease with vigilant monitoring for emergence of infection. However, no definitive conclusion can be drawn from this current level of evidence and prospective trials with well defined protocols are required to define the role of corticosteroids in the treatment of SJS/TEN.

4.10.3. Intravenous Immunoglobulin (IVIg)

The rationale for the use of IVIg was based on its ability in vitro to block Fas and subsequently FasL-mediated apoptosis of keratinocytes [51]. The beneficial role of IVIg in SJS/TEN has been demonstrated in retrospective studies. The largest such study to date comprised 48 patients with TEN with a 44.8% mean TBSA recruited from centres across Europe and the United States. Treatment with IVIg resulted in a more rapid cessation of epidermal detachment and a survival rate of 88%. The authors subsequently recommended a dose of 1 g/kg/daily for 3 days [143]. Studies have also demonstrated benefit when investigators have compared the rates of mortality following the use of IVIg with the pre-treatment estimate using SCORTEN. For example, Campione et al, found that 400 mg/kg/daily for 5 days of IVIg resulted in a mortality rate of 10%, significantly lower that the 35% predicted using SCORTEN [144]. Metry et al, showed that the benefit of IVIg extended to the paediatric population [145].

In 2006, a retrospective study found that the use of IVIg at a total dose of 2.8 g/kg/daily in 23 patients resulted in a marked difference in mortality compared to 8 patients who received supportive therapy alone despite the absence of a difference in SCORTEN between the two groups. The mortality rate was 26% in the patient group receiving IVIg and 75% in the group receiving supportive care only. This difference, however, was not statistically significant. A study by Yang et al, showed a lower than predicted mortality rate for patients given IVIg and corticosteroids and a higher than expected mortality rate for those receiving corticosteroids alone. This difference was not statistically significant [146].

Despite the initial preponderance of evidence favouring the use of IVIG in SJS/TEN, a few published reports have not demonstrated any benefit. Most of these studies comparing the use of IVIg with supportive care alone used doses less than the recommended 2-3 g/kg [147]-[150]. The largest restrospective analysis on the use of IVIg derived from the EuroSCAR study and published in 2008 included 109 patients with TEN, 136 with SJS/TEN overlap, and 134 with SJS found that IVIg administered at a dose of 1.9 g/kg conferred an OR of 1.4 when compared to the use of supportive measures alone. This study involved the use of lower than recommended doses of IVIg and the patients from the IVIg group tended to have a greater TBSA involvement [151]. A controlled observational study in an intensive care unit in a French dermatology department of 34 patients who presented at a mean of 4.3 days after the onset of TEN revealed a higher mortality rate than that predicted by SCORTEN when 2g/kg of IVIg was administered within 2 days of admission [85].

Randomized control studies are required using sufficient doses of IVIg to characterize its benefit in not only reducing mortality but also arresting the rate of progression and hastening the rate of re-epithelialization. However, the evidence thus far, is not robust as an adjunctive immunomodulatory therapy in the treatment of SJS/TEN.

4.10.4. C yclosporine

Cyclosporine inhibits CD8 activation and subsequent release of granulysin, granzyme and perforin as well as inhibiting the proapoptotic effect of NF-κB. Several case and case series reports have shown arrest of disease progression and shorter time to re-epithelialization with doses varying from 3-10 mg/kg/daily for a period ranging from 8 days to several weeks [152] [153]-[161]. The study by Arevalo et al, showed that outcomes for 10 patients treated with cyclosporin was superior to 6 patients treated with cyclophosphamide and corticosteroids with respect to re-epithelialization, disease progression and death [157]. However, randomized control studies are required to better define its benefits, the appropriate dose and duration of therapy. Furthermore, no studies have been published to date evaluating the efficacy of using both IVIg and cyclosporine but may be worthwhile considering as different pathways involved in the pathogenesis of SJS/TEN are targeted.

4.10.5. Plasmapheresis

Plasmapheresis (PE) has been reported to be beneficial in several case reports and series in patients with TEN based on the principle that the drug, drug metabolite or cytotoxic mediator is removed from the circulation [162]-[165]. One report from Sweden showed no benefit from PE in eight patients compared with patients from other studies who received similar support

http://dx.doi.org/10.5772/54820

care but without PE [166]. There is insufficient evidence at this stage to support the use of PE in preference to other adjunctive measures.

4.10.6. Anti-TNF therapy

TNF is thought to be upregulated in TEN and immunohistochemistry has demonstrated increased levels of TNF from 23 patients as compared with controls [167]. Thalidomide, a potent inhibitor of TNF, was found in a double blinded randomized placebo controlled trial to be lethal in 10 of 12 patients compared with 3 of 10 control subjects. The exact mechanism underlying these fatalities is unknown but the drug is firmly contraindicated in SJS/TEN.

Infliximab and eternecept has been shown to be beneficial in a small number of case reports [168]-[173]. The drug was usually administered late in the course of disease and therefore its benefit is not clear and requires case-control studies to further elucidate its role.

4.10.7. N-acetylcysteine

Strategies have been explored to overcome the diminished detoxifying capacity of abnormal inherent metabolic pathways evident in a proportion of patients with SJS/TEN. Administration of N-acetylcysteine enhances the oxidant buffering capacity of glutathione, which enhances the detoxification of a range of drugs, as well as inhibiting NF-κB. Two case reports have shown a beneficial response but larger studies are clearly required before it is readily applied in clinical practice [174],[175].

4.10.8. Restricted use of related medications

In addition to the restricted use of the same medication, structurally similar drugs should also be avoided. The aromatic anticonvulsants carbamazepine, phenytoin and phenobarbitol cross react with one another. Cross reactivity resulting in SJS/TEN can also occur across different classes of beta-lactam antibiotics, such as penicillins, cephalosporins and carbapenems [176]. Administration of a structurally related drug can also result in different reactions. One case report described a patient with ceftriaxone-induced TEN who developed immediate anaphylaxis following the administration of piperacillin/tazobactam [177].

The risk of SJS/TEN with structurally distinct agents within the same class of drug is less clear. For example, the cross reactivity between a priopionic acid NSAID and an enolic acid NSAID is unknown. The safest practice is to restrict all NSAIDs following NSAID-induced SJS/TEN.

5. Drug induced hypersensitivity syndrome

5.1. Nosology

The term hypersensitivity syndrome has been used for decades to describe a cutaneous drug reaction accompanied by involvement of internal organs. In 1938, Merritt and Putnam described a toxic reaction to phenytoin characterized by exfoliative dermatitis, fever and eosinophilia [178]. This was distinguished from those patients who developed a mild, morbilliform rash. Chaiken et al coined the term Dilantin hypersensitivity in 1950 to further characterize the systemic reaction described by Merritt and Putnam to also include lymphadenopathy and multivisceral involvement [179]. Saltzein in 1959 described a drug-induced lymphoma characterized by lymphadenopathy and diffuse skin nodules and plaques without internal organ involvement. [180]. The anticonvulsant hypersensitivity syndrome was named in 1988 by Shear and Spielberg to refer the similar cutaneous and systemic manifestations of idiosyncratic reactions to a range of anticonvulsant medications including phenytoin, phenobarbitol and carbamazepine [181]. In 1996, Bocquet et al introduced the term drug reaction with eosinophilia and systemic symptoms (DRESS) to distinguish it from drug-induced pseudolymphoma and other drug reactions that are not associated with eosinophilia [182]. Finally, Shiohara et al proposed the term drug induced hypersensitivity syndrome (DIHS) to include patients who may not have marked eosinophilia but have other evidence of leukocyte abnormalities, internal organ involvement and evidence of HHV-6 reactivation [183],[184].

5.2. Epidemiology

The incidence of DIHS is estimated to be between 1 in 1000 and 1 in 10000 to phenytoin [185]. The true incidence remains to be determined because of the variable presentations and the lack of universally accepted criteria. The JSCAR and RegiSCAR studies will provide more accurate reporting on the basis of stringent criteria. Preliminary data from the RegiSCAR study suggests that it affects males and females equally with a mean age of 47.4 years (range 3-84 years) [186].

5.3. Etiology and clinical features

Various diagnostic criteria have been proposed. Bocquet et al stipulated the presence of (1) cutaneous drug eruption; (2) hematologic abnormalities including eosinophilia greater than 1.5 $x10^9/L$ or the presence of atypical lymphocytes; and (3) systemic involvement including adenopathy greater than 2 cm in diameter, hepatitis (liver transaminase values >2 normal), interstitial nephritis, interstitial pneumonia, or carditis.

Kardaun et al developed a scoring system to validate the diagnosis [187].

The potential role of HHV-6 in the pathogenesis of DIHS was incorporated into the criteria for DIHS by the JSCAR group [188]: (1) maculopapular rash developing more than 3 weeks after starting a limited number of drugs; (2) prolonged clinical symptoms 2 weeks after discontinuation of the causative drug; (3) fever greater than 38 C; (4) liver abnormalities (eg, ALT levels >100 U/L); (5) leukocyte abnormalities such as leukocytosis (>11 x $10^9/L$), atypical lymphocytosis (>5%), and/or eosinophilia (>1.5 109/L); (6) lymphadenopathy; and (7) HHV-6 reactivation. Diagnosis of typical DIHS requires the presence of all 7 criteria. If criteria 1-5 are present only, then a diagnosis of atypical DIHS is made.

The syndrome typically begins 3 weeks to 3months after commencing therapy with a limited number of drugs of which the most prominent ones are listed below.

http://dx.doi.org/10.5772/54820

Assessment/Score	-1	0	1	2	min	max
Fever ≥38.5°C	n	y			-1	0
Enlarged lymph nodes		n/u	y		0	1
Eosinophilia						
Eosinophilia		n/u	700-1499/μL	"/>1500/μL	0	2
Eosinophilia if WCC<4000/μL			10-19.9%	≥20%		
Atyical lymphocytes		n/u	y		0	1
Skin involvement						
Skin rash extent (%TBSA)		n/u	"/>50%			
Skin rash suggestive of DRESS	n	u	y		-2	2
Histology suggestive of DRESS	n	y/u				
Organ involvement *						
Liver						
Kidney						
Lung		n/u	"/>1 y	≥2 y	0	2
Heart						
Pancreas						
Other organ						
Resolution ≥15 days	n	y			-1	0
Serology/PCR Hepatitis A,B,C EBV,CMV Mycoplasma,Chlamydia ANA Blood culture						
If non +ve and ≥3 -ve				n	0	1
Total					-4	9

y, yes; n, no.

*After exclusion of other causes: 0, no organ involvement; 1, 1 organ involved; 2, ≥ 2 organs involved.

Final score: <2, excluded; 2-3, possible; 4-5, probable; >5, definite.

Table 3. Diagnostic validation score for DRESS

High-grade fever (38-40°C) is usually the first symptom followed by the development of facial oedema (Fig. 8), often with pinhead-sized pustules, and an erythroderma with edematous, follicular and purpuric lesions (Fig. 9). An exfoliative dermatitis often eventuates especially if

Carbamazepine
Phenytoin
Phenobarbitol
Zonisamide
Lamotrigine
Allopurinol
Dapsone
Sulphasalazine
Mexiletine
Minocycline
Strontium ranelate
Abacavir

Table 4. The main causative drugs of DIHS

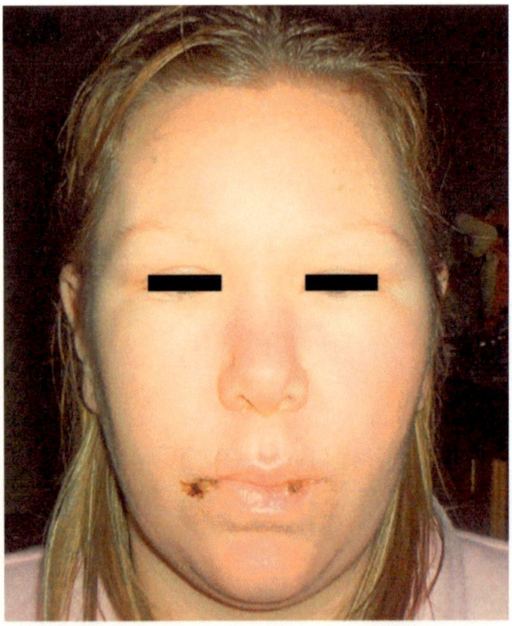

Figure 8. Facial erythema and edema with labial ulceration in a young woman with DIHS/DRESS.

the causative drug is not withdrawn (Fig. 10). Cheilitis (Fig. 8), pharyngeal erythema and oral ulceration may occur but severe stomatitis is not present. Tender lymphadenopathy in more than two sites and bilateral swelling of salivary glands with xerostomia is evident early in the course of disease. Hepatosplenomegaly is a common finding. Leukocytosis with atypical lymphocytes and eosinophilia (60-70% of cases) is a prominent feature of this syndrome although the eosinophilia may not be observed for 1-2 weeks. Thrombocytopenia and anemia may also be present. Hypogammaglobulinema is noted at the onset of disease with the nadir occurring several days after the withdrawal of the causative drug [189]. An overshoot in the IgG level occurs 1-2 weeks after the nadir before returning to normal on full recovery. Internal organ involvement is listed in table 5.

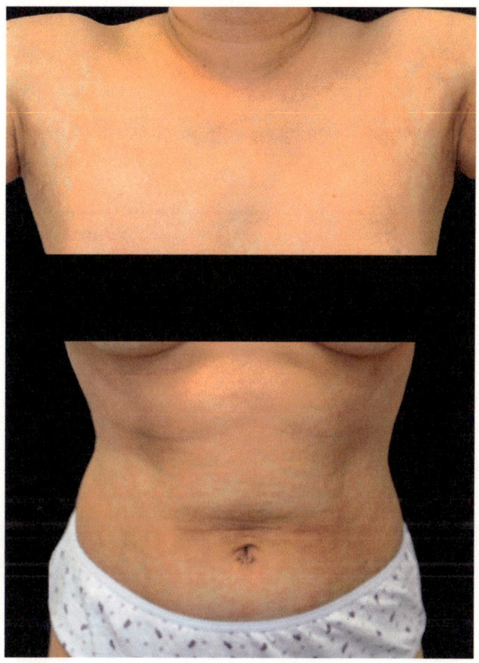

Figure 9. Maculopapular eruption and erythroderma of the trunk in DIHS.

The onset of symptoms is variable with patients developing 2-3 symptomatic features followed by stepwise development of other manifestations. In most cases, withdrawal of the drug is not followed by rapid resolution of symptoms. Many patients may continue to deteriorate and show periodic relapses for weeks after the withdrawal of the causative drug.

Several reports have described the occurrence of autoantibody formation and autoimmune diseases up to 4 years after the acute resolution of DIHS/DRESS [201] and these include type 1 diabetes mellitus [202], autoimmune thyroid disease [203], scleroderma GVHD [204], SLE [205], and bullous pemphigoid [206]. One of the likely explanations for the occurrence of autoimmune disease is the depletion of regulatory T cells upon recovery of disease.

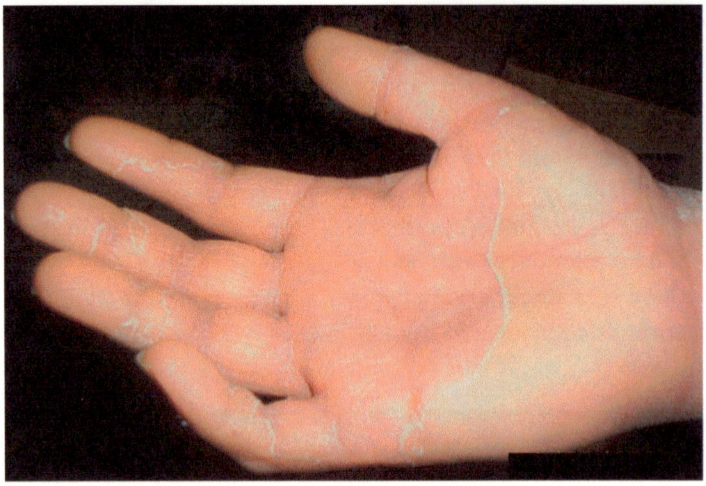

Figure 10. Exfoliative dermatitis involving the hand in a young woman with DIHS/DRESS who had continued to ingest the culprit drug for 4 weeks when this image was taken.

Manifestation	Comments
Hepatitis (mixed hepatocellular and cholestatic)	71%[190]
Interstitial nephritis	11%, frequent with Allopurinol-induced DIHS[191]
Pneumonitis/pleuritis	Common in minocycline[192] and abacavir[193] induced DIHS
Myocarditis	Occurs at onset or 40 days after onset of DIHS[194]
Limbic encephalitis	2-4 weeks after onset of DIHS, HHV-6 reactivation in CSF[195] May be assoiciated with SiADH[196]
CMV Gastrointestinal ulceration with bleeding	4-5 weeks after onset of DIHS[197]
Haemaophagocytic syndrome	Rare, occurs 2 weeks after onset of disease[198]
Parotid gland enlargement	Rare[199]
Pancreatitis	Rare[200]

Table 5. Internal organ involvement in DIHS

Abacavir, an HIV nucleoside analogue reverse transcriptase inhibitor causes a potentially life-threatening hypersensitivity syndrome in approximately 5-8% of recipients within 6 weeks of therapy [207],[208]. The clinical and laboratory features of this syndrome differs from typical cases of DIHS/DRESS in that there is a predilection for the gastrointestinal system with nausea, abdominal pain, diarrhoea, and the respiratory tract with cough, pharyngitis and shortness of breath. Headache, myalgia and/or arthralgia may also be present. Eosinophilia is present in < 10% of cases and liver function test abnormalities are detected in < 20% of cases [209]. Also, the manifestations resolve within 72 hours rather than having a protracted relapsing course and the role of herpetic viruses in this condition is unknown.

5.4. Differential diagnosis

Viral infections such as EBV, CMV, and measles can be distinguished by the absence of eosinophilia, hypogammaglobulinemia, and supportive serology. In children, DIHS/DRESS is differentiated from Kawasaki's disease by the absence of a bulbar conjunctivitis, strawberry tongue, coronary aneurysms, hypoalbuminemia and thrombocytosis. Serum sickness is characterized by urticarial lesions and the absence of internal organ involvement. Atopic erythroderma with bacterial infection does not usually involve hepatitis or nephritis. Drug-induced pseudolymphoma from carbamazepine or phenytoin is distinguished from DIHS/DRESS by the absence of internal organ involvement and the prompt resolution of symptoms when the drug is withdrawn. Cutaneous B and T cell lymphomas have an indolent course and characteristic histopathology.

5.5. Pathology

The histopathology of DIHS/DRESS is relatively non-specific and consists of a lymphocytic infiltrate that is superficial, perivascular, dense and diffuse. Eosinophils may be present but is often absent. The presence of loose rather than discrete granulomatous aggregates of histiocytes have been recently reported (Figs. 11, 12) [210]. This may be due to continued exposure to the culprit drug after the onset of DIHS/DRESS. Granuloma formation occurs as a consequence of a delayed-type hypersensitivity (type IV) reaction, the classic example of which is the tuberculin reaction where a cutaneous granuloma is induced after injection of purified protein derivative in a previously sensitized individual. The expansion of CD4 cells and the secretion of IFN-γ and other Th-1 cytokines result in the recruitment of macrophages. Sustained drug exposure and the persistence of cytokine release promote differentiation of macrophages into epithelioid cells, which secrete TNF promoting their fusion to form multinucleate giant cells and granulomas. HHV-6 and DNA from other herpes viruses may be detected in skin lesions by PCR or in situ hybridization [183].

5.6. Drug allergy testing

5.6.1. Patch tests

Santiago et al recently studied the utility of patch testing in DIHS/DRESS and found a positive reaction in 32% of the 56 patients. Patch testing was performed between 6 weeks and 6 months after healing of the lesion and at least one month after corticosteroids were ceased. They found that 76% of the 17 patients with carbamazepine-induced DIHS/DRESS were patch test positive but none of the 19 allopurinol-sensitive patients were positive to allopurinol and its metabolite, oxypurinol. No systemic reactions occurred during or after testing [211]. Hence patch testing may prove useful once the reagent and timing of such testing is optimized. Patch testing has,

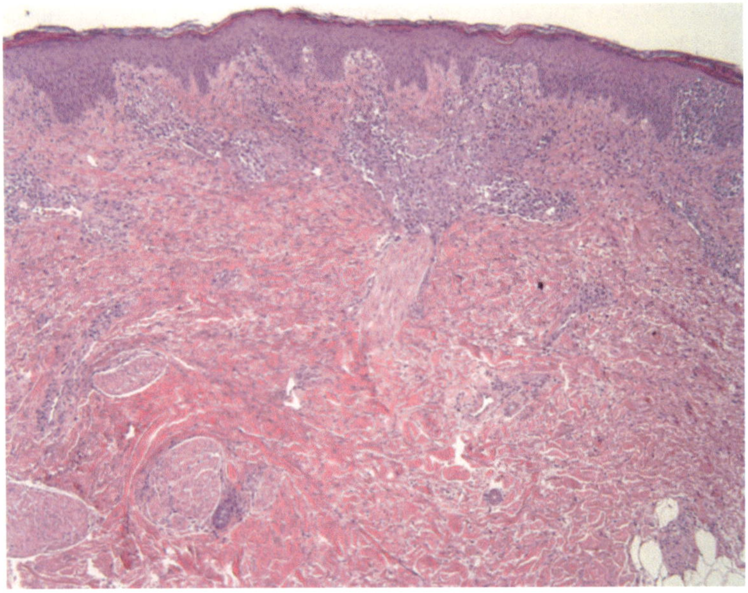

Figure 11. Low power view of a skin biopsy from a patient with DIHS demonstrating the superficial dermal nature and perivascular distribution of the inflammatory infiltrate with acanthosis and hyperkeratosis of the epidermis (Hematoxylin-eosin, original magnification x40).

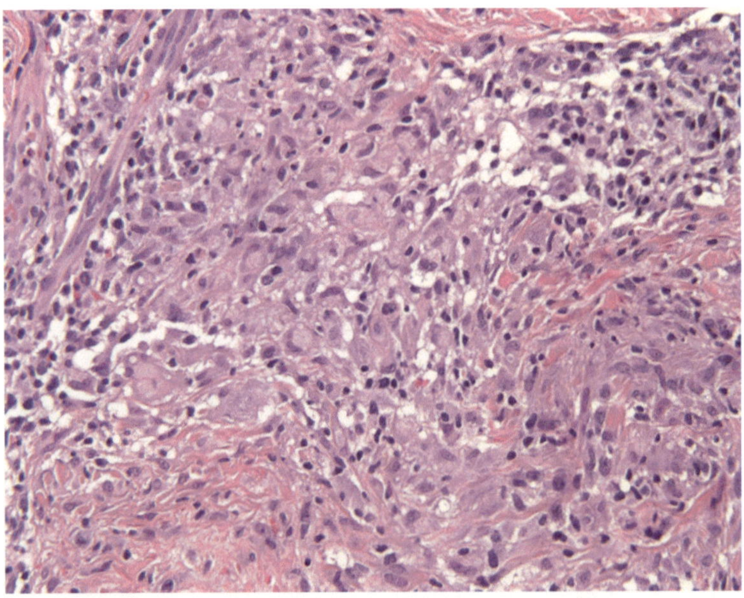

Figure 12. High power view of a skin biopsy from a patient with DIHS demonstrates granulomatous inflammation with prominent, but relatively loosely aggregated histiocytes, mixed with lymphocytes. Eosinophils are absent (Hematoxylin-eosin, original magnification x200).

however, proven to be very useful in confirming suspected cases for abacavir hypersensitivity with a higher degree of specificity than can be confirmed clinically [212].

5.6.2. Lymphocyte transformation tests(LTTs)

LTTs are usually negative up to 3 weeks after the onset of DIHS/DRESS but most patients are positive at 5-7 weeks and have persistent responses even at 1 year. Treatment with corticosteroids did not affect the results [97]. One possible explanation for the negative LTT result during the acute phase of DIHS is the expansion T regulatory cells with a naïve phenotype (CD4CD25FoxP3), which then are depleted by apoptosis during the recovery phase. These regulatory T cells are capable of suppressing proliferation of memory T cells in LTTs [55].

5.7. Pathogenesis

The pathogenesis of DIHS/DRESS is still to be fully elucidated. The precise role of HHV-6 in DIHS is unclear. The initiating event may be the reactivation of one or more herpetic viruses, which is clinically unapparent. Virus-stimulated T cells may then cross react with drug-derived hapten-protein conjugates that are presented by dendritic cells to naïve antigen-specific CD4 T-cells with the subsequent differentiation into effector/memory CD4 cells. These dendritic cells may also activate CD8 T-cells by cross-presentation. The expansion of effector CD4 T-cells with their production of IFN-γ and other cytokines results in recruitment and activation of macrophages. Failure to eradicate the antigenic stimulus, in this instance due to the continued ingestion of the drug, causes persistent cytokine release and promotes differentiation of macrophages into epithelioid cells, which secrete large amounts of TNF promoting their fusion to form multinucleate giant cells [210]. Analogous to that observed in GVHD, longitudinal real-time PCR analyses of viral loads in blood samples drawn from patients with DIHS show that various herpetic viruses are sequentially activated as a result of massive T cell stimulation, B cell loss and hypogammaglobulinemia [213]; Activation of Epstein-Barr virus or HHV-6 extends to the sequential activation of HHV-7, cytomegalovirus and varicella-zoster virus [189]. The frequent deterioration or several exacerbations that occur despite continuation of the drug may at least be partly explained by sequential reactivation of herpetic viruses and the immune response to viral replication. An alternative explanation is that drug specific T cells are activated resulting in reactivation of the viral genome and sequential reactivation of herpes viruses.

Genetic susceptibility may also play a role as all patients with allopurinol-induced DIHS in a Han Chinese population harboured the *HLA-B*5801* allele compared with 15% of control subjects [67]. Recently, an association was described between *HLA-A*3101* and DIHS in Northern Europeans; OR 12.41 [1.27-121.03] [64] and in the Japanese; OR 9.5 [4.6–19.5] [65]. In a Western Australian HIV Cohort Study, *HLA-B*5701* was present in 14 (78%) of the 18 patients with abacavir hypersensitivity, and in four (2%) of the 167 abacavir tolerant patients; OR 117 [29-481] [193]. There is a discrepancy in the association of *HLA-B*5701* and abacavir hypersensitivity across various racial groups The association was confirmed in a separate cohort of HIV-infected white Americans and was also found to confer susceptibility in Hispanics but not in blacks [214]. No association was found in a cohort of Korean patients [215]. Hence screening for *HLA-B*5701* is not useful in predicting sensitivity in all patients. The racial variation may be partly explained by the differences in MHC haplotypes across different racial groups. The Caucasian 57.1 ancestral haplotype, which confers susceptibility to abacavir hypersensitivity possibly as a result of strong linkage disequilibrium with other candidate genetic factors such as cellular chaperones (e.g. heat shock proteins), inflammatory cytokines (e.g. TNF), and proteins involved in the stress response (e.g. MHC class I chain-related genes, MIC-A and MIC-B). African populations do not demonstrate this haplotype [216]. However, in a recent study by Saag et al, all 42 white patients with immunologically confirmed (i.e. positive patch tests) hypersensitivity reactions were *HLA-B*5701* positive (sensitivity 100%, OR 1945 [110-34,352]) but in addition all 5 black patients with immunologically confirmed hypersensitivity reactions were *HLA-B*5701* positive (sensitivity 100%, OR 900 [38-21,045]. Screening for the *HLA-B*5701* has eliminated immunologically confirmed cases of abacavir hypersensitivity [217].

5.8. Treatment

Early recognition of the syndrome with cessation of the causative drug is essential in improving patient outcomes. No randomized controlled trials have been conducted to determine the appropriate adjunctive therapy for DIHS/DRESS. Oral corticosteroids at 1 mg/kg/daily is commenced and tapered over at least 6-8 weeks to prevent relapse of various cutaneous and visceral manifestations of the syndrome. If symptoms deteriorate despite corticosteroid therapy then IVIg [218],[219], plasma exchange [220], rituximab, gangciclovir or a combination of these modalities [221] can be considered.

Recently, the French Society of Dermatology formulated guidelines on the management of DIHS/DRESS [133]:

1. Absence of signs of severity: topical corticosteroids, emollients and H1-antihistamines.
2. Presence of signs of severity (transaminases >5 times normal, renal impairment, pneumonia, hemophagocytosis, cardiac involvement): prednisone 1 mg/kg/day.
3. Life-threatening signs: (hemophagocytosis with bone marrow failure, encephalitis, severe hepatitis, renal failure, respiratory failure): prednisone and IVIg 2 g/kg over 5 days.
4. Presence of signs of severity with confirmation of major viral reactivation: prednisone and gangciclovir and/or IVIg.

6. Acute generalized exanthematous pustulosis

6.1. Nosology

In 1980, Beylot et al [222] introduced the term acute generalized exanthematous pustulosis (AGEP) to describe acute pustular reactions with distinct clinical and histological features thereby differentiating it from pustular psoriasis.

6.2. Epidemiology

AGEP is rare with an incidence of 1-5 cases per million per year [223]. The EuroSCAR study comprising 97 validated cases of AGEP recruited from Austria, France, Israel, Italy and the Netherlands, revealed a mean age (±SD) of 56 (±21) years and a female preponderance with a male/female ratio of 0.8 [18]. The predominance in women was shown to be even greater in case series reports from Taiwan (68.7% of 16 cases) [224], and Israel (76.9% of 13 cases) [225]. AGEP has been reported in children, with the largest pediatric series of 20 cases from China [226].

6.3. Clinical features

The clinical manifestations are characterized by fever and a pruritic or burning edematous erythema (Figs. 13 A&B) followed by the rapid appearance of dozens of small (< 5 mm) non-follicular sterile pustules (Fig. 14). The skin lesions are often accentuated in the intertriginous areas (Fig. 13 C). There is usually an accompanying marked neutrophilia (7 x 10^9/L) and in a third of cases, a mild eosinophilia. A mild non-erosive mucous membrane involvement occurs in 20% of cases. Internal organ involvement is uncommon and usually is confined to a slight reduction in creatinine clearance and mild elevation of aminotransferases.

The clinical course is characterized by spontaneous resolution of skin and systemic manifestations over a period of up to 15 days once the offending agent is withdrawn [223]. AGEP has a favourable prognosis; the reported mortality rate is up to 5% and poor outcomes usually result from secondary infection in the elderly or those patients with significant comorbidities [227],[228].

6.4. Etiology

AGEP is caused by drugs in at least 90% of cases. According to the EuroSCAR study, the agents conferring the highest risk are pristinamycin, aminopenicillins, hydroxychloroquine, antibacterial sulphonamides, terbinafine and diltiazem [18]. The latent period is short (usually 1-5 days) with the EuroScar study demonstrating that it may vary for different drugs. For antibiotics, including sulphonamides, the median latent period was 1 day, and for other drugs it was 11 days [18].

Contact sensitivity has been implicated in a few case reports. Causative agents include mercury[229], and bufexemac, a potent topical NSAID[230]. Neither of these agents was implicated in the 97 cases of AGEP in the EuroScar. The role of infectious agents in AGEP has been suggested in various case reports due to the absence of an inciting drug [231]. The organisms include coxsackie B4 [232], cytomegalovirus [233], parvovirus B19 [234], *Chlamydia pneumoniae* [235], and *Escherichia coli* [236]. No significant risk for infection was found in the EuroScar study although the study was not designed to identify potential causative organisms. Spider bites were suggested as a cause AGEP in a series of three cases from Israel, presumably as a result of the venom's ability to induce IL-8 and GM-CSF [237]. Finally, as illustrated in two recent cases, AGEP may develop without preceding medication or disease [238].

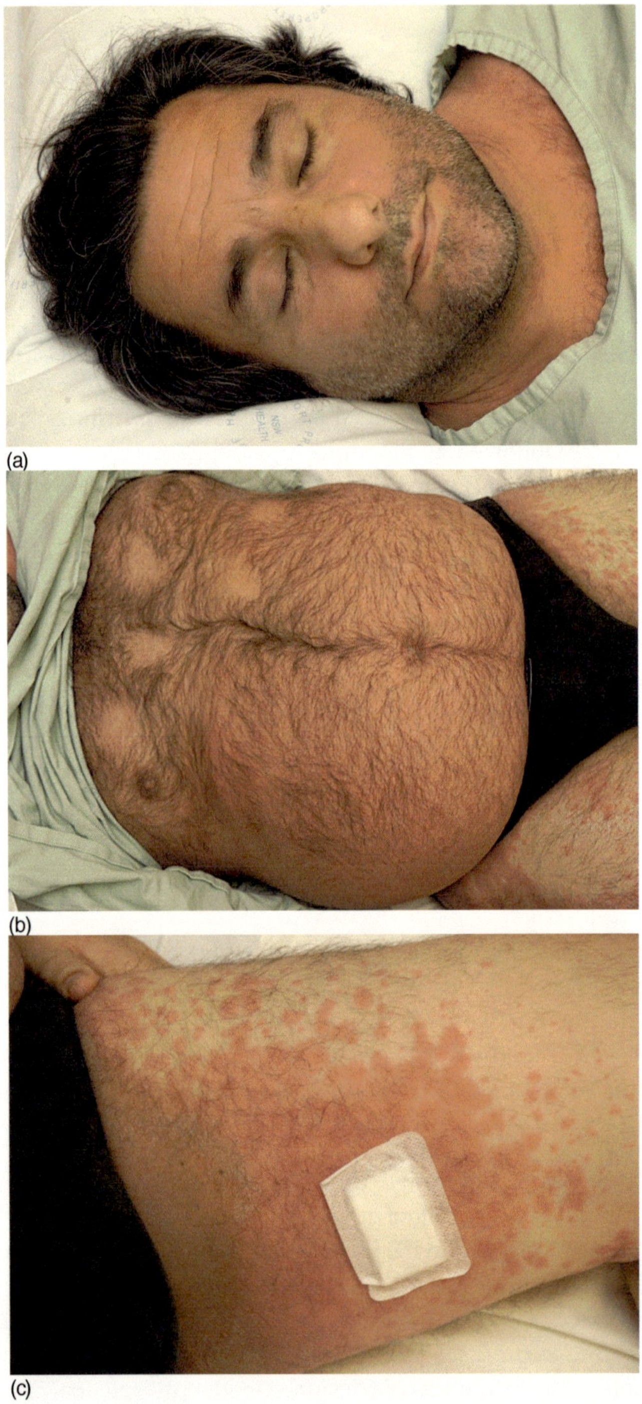

Figure 13. This patient with AGEP had an onset of erythema and edema of the face (A), erythema of the trunk (B) with a predilection for intertriginous areas (C).

http://dx.doi.org/10.5772/54820

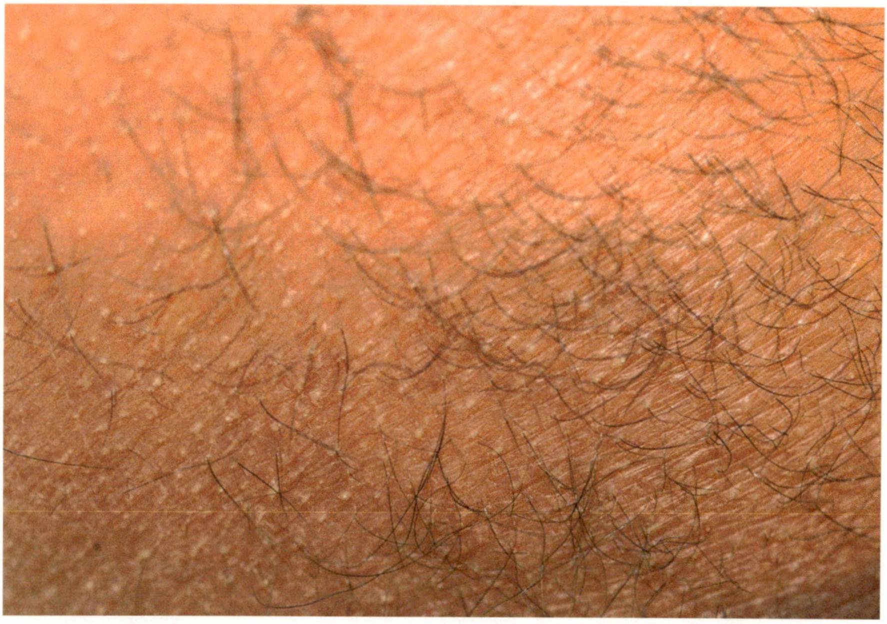

Figure 14. The lesions of AGEP occur rapidly and are characterized by dozens of small (< 5 mm) non-follicular sterile pustules.

6.5. Pathogenesis

The pathogenesis of AGEP has been elucidated by patch [239],[240] and in vitro tests [241]-[243] and initially involves activation, expansion and subsequent migration of drug-specific CD4 and CD8 cells to the skin. The initial influx of CD8 cytotoxic T cells results in apoptosis of keratinocytes and the formation of subcorneal vesicles. The infiltrating CD4 cells release CXCL-8, which results in recruitment of neutrophils, and granulocyte macrophage-colony stimulating factor (GM-CSF), which prevents apoptosis of neutrophils. This results in the conversion of vesicles into pustules. CD4 cells also release IFN-γ, which stimulates keratinocytes to secrete CXCL-8, as well as RANTES and IL-5, which contributes to the eosinophilia observed in some patients [244]. Resident Langerhans' cells may present drug antigens to CD4 cells and keratinocytes may act as antigen presenting cells to CD8 cells thereby augmenting the neutrophil-mediated inflammatory response. Genetic susceptibility to AGEP has not been robustly examined and therefore remains largely unknown.

6.6. Diagnostic tests

A pustular smear should be performed to exclude an infectious aetiology. A full blood count will reveal a neutrophilia. A skin biopsy may show (spongiform or non-spongiform) subcorneal and/or intradermal pustules, edema of the papillary dermis, perivascular infiltrates with neutrophils and exocytosis of some eosinophils and focal necrotic keratinocytes (Fig. 15). The typical changes of psoriasis such as acanthosis and papillomatosis are usually absent. Patch testing may be useful in confirming the association between AGEP and the culprit drugs. In a controlled study, patch tests were positive in half of the 14 cases of AGEP [96]. Readings should not be restricted to 24 and 48 hours after the application of the drug but should also be determined at 96 and 120 hours to maximise sensitivity. Pustule formation is often observed in positive patch tests in cases of AGEP. The test can be conducted one month after resolution of the disease. The risk of AGEP with patch testing is considered to be low but not negligible [245]. A small number of studies have supported a role for LTT [246], IFN-γ release [247], lymphokine macrophage migration inhibition factor release assays [241] but these in vitro tests are not widely available and its value remains to be determined in large cohorts.

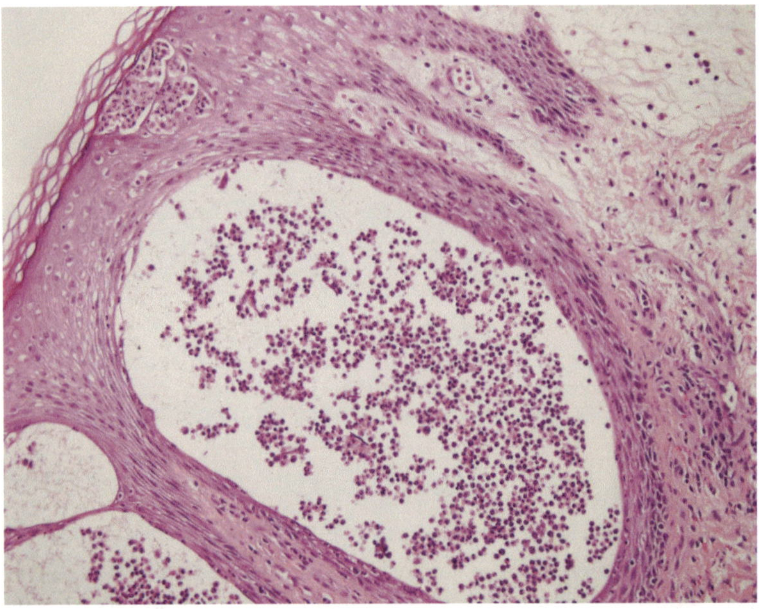

Figure 15. A moderate power view of a skin biopsy from a patient with AGEP shows spongiform subcorneal pustules, edema of the papillary dermis and perivascular infiltrates with neutrophils and exocytosis of some eosinophils.

Morphology **Pustules**	
Typical	+2
Compatible with disease	+1
Insufficient	0
Erythema	
Typical	+2
Compatible with disease	+1
Insufficient	0
Distribution	

http://dx.doi.org/10.5772/54820

Morphology	
Pustules	
Typical	+2
Compatible with disease	+1
Insufficient	0
Post pustular desquamation	
Yes	+1
No	0
Course	
Mucous membrane involvement	
Yes	-2
No	0
Acute onset	
Yes	0
No	-2
Resolution	
Yes	0
No	-4
Fever ≥ 38°C	
Yes	+1
No	0
Polymorphonuclear cells ≥ 7/µl	
Yes	+1
No	0
Histology	
Other disease	-10
Not representative	0
Exocytosis of polymorphonuclear cells	+1
Subcorneal and/or intraepidermal non-spongiform pustules or NOS pustules with papillary edema or subcorneal and/or intraepidermal spongiform pustulea or NOS pustules without papillary edema	+2
Spongiform subcorneal and/or intraepidermal pustules with papillary edema	+3

NOS, not otherwise specified.

Score ≤ 0; excluded, 1-4: possible, 5-7: probable, 8-12: definite

Table 6. Diagnostic score for validation of AGEP

6.7. Differential diagnosis

AGEP, which is characterized by non-follicular pustules can be readily distinguished from diseases with follicular pustulosis such as bacterial folliculitis, furunculosis, acneiform eruptions, pustular contact dermatitis, dermatophyte infection, viral exanthema with primary vesiculation and secondary postulation, impetigo, Sweet syndrome and SSSS. Other diseases are not as easily differentiated from AGEP. Generalized pustular psoriasis (Zumbusch psoriasis) is characterized by pustules that slowly develop on areas of psoriasis accompanied by the histological changes of psoriasis on skin biopsy. There is also usually a family history of psoriasis. Sneddon-Wilkinson disease (subcorneal pustulosis) and subcorneal IgA dermatosis are characterized by the subacute development of larger pustules than those that erupt in AGEP and maybe associated with hyopyon formation.

A diagnostic score was devised to validate the diagnosis of AGEP based on the morphology, course of disease, and histology and assist in the differentiation from similar diseases [223].

6.8. Treatment

As AGEP is a self-limiting disease with a favourable prognosis. Cessation of the causative agent and supportive treatment is usually all that his required. In the pustular phase, supportive measures consist of moist dressings with drying and disinfecting solutions to avoid superinfection. In the postpustular desquamation phase, emollients are used to optimise preservation of skin barrier function. In a study of nine cases from Israel, all of who made a full recovery, seven received supportive care alone and the other two received corticosteroids [248]. It remains to be established whether oral or parenteral corticosteroids hasten the resolution of disease. A brief course of systemic corticosteroids may be considered in patients with severe and widespread inflammation of the skin.

7. Conclusion

SCARs such as SJS/TEN, DIHS/DRESS, and AGEP are idiosyncratic and specific types of reactions that have distinct clinical, laboratory and histological features. The definition of DIHS/DRESS has not been universally adopted and will need to be clarified once the role of herpetic viruses and characteristic histological features are known. The early identification of these reactions and the subsequent prompt withdrawal of therapy and the implementation of supportive and adjunctive therapies are crucial in minimising morbidity and rates of mortality. Multicentre randomized studies are required to adopt the most suitable therapies for these potentially life-threatening conditions. The emergence in the understanding of HLA susceptibility genes will enable patients to be screened for the risk of developing a SCAR and will hopefully be more widely performed once cost effective and rapid methods of detection are widely available to the prescribing doctor.

http://dx.doi.org/10.5772/54820

Author details

Suran L. Fernando[1,2]

1 Department of Clinical Immunology and Allergy, Royal North Shore Hospital, Sydney, Australia

2 Sydney Medical School – Northern, Sydney University, Sydney, Australia

References

[1] von Hebra F. Acute exantheme und hautkrankheiten. *Handbuch der Speciellen Pathologie und Therapie* 1860:198-200.

[2] Stevens AM, Johnson FC. A new eruptive fever associated with stomatitis and ophthalmia: report of two cases in children. *Am J Dis Child* 1922;24:526-533.

[3] Thomas BA. The so-called Stevens-Johnson syndrome. *Br Med J* 1950;1(4667):1393-7.

[4] Lyell A. Toxic epidermal necrolysis: an eruption resembling scalding of the skin. *Br J Dermatol* 1956;68(11):355-61.

[5] Ruiz-Maldonado R. Acute disseminated epidermal necrosis types 1, 2, and 3: study of sixty cases. *J Am Acad Dermatol* 1985;13(4):623-35.

[6] Lyell A. Requiem for toxic epidermal necrolysis. *Br J Dermatol* 1990;122(6):837-8.

[7] Bastuji-Garin S, Rzany B, Stern RS, Shear NH, Naldi L, Roujeau JC. Clinical classification of cases of toxic epidermal necrolysis, Stevens-Johnson syndrome, and erythema multiforme. *Arch Dermatol* 1993;129(1):92-6.

[8] Kokuba H, Imafuku S, Huang S, Aurelian L, Burnett JW. Erythema multiforme lesions are associated with expression of a herpes simplex virus (HSV) gene and qualitative alterations in the HSV-specific T-cell response. *Br J Dermatol* 1998;138(6):952-64.

[9] Villiger RM, von Vigier RO, Ramelli GP, Hassink RI, Bianchetti MG. Precipitants in 42 cases of erythema multiforme. *Eur J Pediatr* 1999;158(11):929-32.

[10] Ng PP, Sun YJ, Tan HH, Tan SH. Detection of herpes simplex virus genomic DNA in various subsets of Erythema multiforme by polymerase chain reaction. *Dermatology* 2003;207(4):349-53.

[11] Mockenhaupt M, Viboud C, Dunant A, et al. Stevens-Johnson syndrome and toxic epidermal necrolysis: assessment of medication risks with emphasis on recently marketed drugs. The EuroSCAR-study. *J Invest Dermatol* 2008;128(1):35-44.

[12] Carrozzo M, Togliatto M, Gandolfo S. [Erythema multiforme. A heterogeneous pathologic phenotype]. *Minerva Stomatol* 1999;48(5):217-26.

[13] Lam NS, Yang YH, Wang LC, Lin YT, Chiang BL. Clinical characteristics of childhood erythema multiforme, Stevens-Johnson syndrome and toxic epidermal necrolysis in Taiwanese children. *J Microbiol Immunol Infect* 2004;37(6):366-70.

[14] Cote B, Wechsler J, Bastuji-Garin S, Assier H, Revuz J, Roujeau JC. Clinicopathologic correlation in erythema multiforme and Stevens-Johnson syndrome. *Arch Dermatol* 1995;131(11):1268-72.

[15] Rzany B, Mockenhaupt M, Baur S, et al. Epidemiology of erythema exsudativum multiforme majus, Stevens-Johnson syndrome, and toxic epidermal necrolysis in Germany (1990-1992): structure and results of a population-based registry. *J Clin Epidemiol* 1996;49(7):769-73.

[16] Kelly JP, Auquier A, Rzany B, et al. An international collaborative case-control study of severe cutaneous adverse reactions (SCAR). Design and methods. *J Clin Epidemiol* 1995;48(9):1099-108.

[17] Roujeau JC, Kelly JP, Naldi L, et al. Medication use and the risk of Stevens-Johnson syndrome or toxic epidermal necrolysis. *N Engl J Med* 1995;333(24):1600-7.

[18] Sidoroff A, Dunant A, Viboud C, et al. Risk factors for acute generalized exanthematous pustulosis (AGEP)-results of a multinational case-control study (EuroSCAR). *Br J Dermatol* 2007;157(5):989-96.

[19] Rzany B, Correia O, Kelly JP, Naldi L, Auquier A, Stern R. Risk of Stevens-Johnson syndrome and toxic epidermal necrolysis during first weeks of antiepileptic therapy: a case-control study. Study Group of the International Case Control Study on Severe Cutaneous Adverse Reactions. *Lancet* 1999;353(9171):2190-4.

[20] Levi N, Bastuji-Garin S, Mockenhaupt M, et al. Medications as risk factors of Stevens-Johnson syndrome and toxic epidermal necrolysis in children: a pooled analysis. *Pediatrics* 2009;123(2):e297-304.

[21] Fournier S, Bastuji-Garin S, Mentec H, Revuz J, Roujeau JC. Toxic epidermal necrolysis associated with Mycoplasma pneumoniae infection. *Eur J Clin Microbiol Infect Dis* 1995;14(6):558-9.

[22] Ball R, Ball LK, Wise RP, Braun MM, Beeler JA, Salive ME. Stevens-Johnson syndrome and toxic epidermal necrolysis after vaccination: reports to the vaccine adverse event reporting system. *Pediatr Infect Dis J* 2001;20(2):219-23.

[23] House RA, Jakubovic H, Wong L, Holness DL. Work-related toxic epidermal necrolysis? *J Occup Med* 1992;34(2):135-9.

[24] Revuz J, Roujeau JC, Guillaume JC, Penso D, Touraine R. Treatment of toxic epidermal necrolysis. Creteil's experience. *Arch Dermatol* 1987;123(9):1156-8.

[25] Letko E, Papaliodis DN, Papaliodis GN, Daoud YJ, Ahmed AR, Foster CS. Stevens-Johnson syndrome and toxic epidermal necrolysis: a review of the literature. *Ann Allergy Asthma Immunol* 2005;94(4):419-36; quiz 436-8, 456.

[26] Lebargy F, Wolkenstein P, Gisselbrecht M, et al. Pulmonary complications in toxic epidermal necrolysis: a prospective clinical study. *Intensive Care Med* 1997;23(12): 1237-44.

[27] Kim MJ, Lee KY. Bronchiolitis obliterans in children with Stevens-Johnson syndrome: follow-up with high resolution CT. *Pediatr Radiol* 1996;26(1):22-5.

[28] Sugimoto Y, Mizutani H, Sato T, Kawamura N, Ohkouchi K, Shimizu M. Toxic epidermal necrolysis with severe gastrointestinal mucosal cell death: a patient who excreted long tubes of dead intestinal epithelium. *J Dermatol* 1998;25(8):533-8.

[29] Atiyeh BS, Dham R, Yassin MF, El-Musa KA. Treatment of toxic epidermal necrolysis with moisture-retentive ointment: a case report and review of the literature. *Dermatol Surg* 2003;29(2):185-8.

[30] Wolkenstein P, Revuz J. Toxic epidermal necrolysis. *Dermatol Clin* 2000;18(3):485-95, ix.

[31] Abood GJ, Nickoloff BJ, Gamelli RL. Treatment strategies in toxic epidermal necrolysis syndrome: where are we at? *J Burn Care Res* 2008;29(1):269-76.

[32] Bastuji-Garin S, Fouchard N, Bertocchi M, Roujeau JC, Revuz J, Wolkenstein P. SCORTEN: a severity-of-illness score for toxic epidermal necrolysis. *J Invest Dermatol* 2000;115(2):149-53.

[33] Guegan S, Bastuji-Garin S, Poszepczynska-Guigne E, Roujeau JC, Revuz J. Performance of the SCORTEN during the first five days of hospitalization to predict the prognosis of epidermal necrolysis. *J Invest Dermatol* 2006;126(2):272-6.

[34] Sekula P, Liss Y, Davidovici B, et al. Evaluation of SCORTEN on a cohort of patients with Stevens-Johnson syndrome and toxic epidermal necrolysis included in the RegiSCAR study. *J Burn Care Res* 2011;32(2):237-45.

[35] Yip LW, Thong BY, Lim J, et al. Ocular manifestations and complications of Stevens-Johnson syndrome and toxic epidermal necrolysis: an Asian series. *Allergy* 2007;62(5): 527-31.

[36] De Rojas MV, Dart JK, Saw VP. The natural history of Stevens Johnson syndrome: patterns of chronic ocular disease and the role of systemic immunosuppressive therapy. *Br J Ophthalmol* 2007;91(8):1048-53.

[37] Shammas MC, Lai EC, Sarkar JS, Yang J, Starr CE, Sippel KC. Management of acute Stevens-Johnson syndrome and toxic epidermal necrolysis utilizing amniotic membrane and topical corticosteroids. *Am J Ophthalmol* 2010;149(2):203-213 e2.

[38] Magina S, Lisboa C, Leal V, Palmares J, Mesquita-Guimaraes J. Dermatological and ophthalmological sequels in toxic epidermal necrolysis. *Dermatology* 2003;207(1):33-6.

[39] Meneux E, Wolkenstein P, Haddad B, Roujeau JC, Revuz J, Paniel BJ. Vulvovaginal involvement in toxic epidermal necrolysis: a retrospective study of 40 cases. *Obstet Gynecol* 1998;91(2):283-7.

[40] Noel JC, Buxant F, Fayt I, Bebusschere G, Parent D. Vulval adenosis associated with toxic epidermal necrolysis. *Br J Dermatol* 2005;153(2):457-8.

[41] Revuz J, Penso D, Roujeau JC, et al. Toxic epidermal necrolysis. Clinical findings and prognosis factors in 87 patients. *Arch Dermatol* 1987;123(9):1160-5.

[42] Kamada N, Kinoshita K, Togawa Y, et al. Chronic pulmonary complications associated with toxic epidermal necrolysis: report of a severe case with anti-Ro/SS-A and a review of the published work. *J Dermatol* 2006;33(9):616-22.

[43] Shah AP, Xu H, Sime PJ, Trawick DR. Severe airflow obstruction and eosinophilic lung disease after Stevens-Johnson syndrome. *Eur Respir J* 2006;28(6):1276-9.

[44] Clayton NA, Kennedy PJ. Management of dysphagia in toxic epidermal necrolysis (TEN) and Stevens-Johnson syndrome (SJS). *Dysphagia* 2007;22(3):187-92.

[45] Pichler WJ, Adam J, Daubner B, Gentinetta T, Keller M, Yerly D. Drug hypersensitivity reactions: pathomechanism and clinical symptoms. *Med Clin North Am* 2010;94(4): 645-64, xv.

[46] Pichler WJ. Direct T-cell stimulations by drugs--bypassing the innate immune system. *Toxicology* 2005;209(2):95-100.

[47] Sanderson JP, Naisbitt DJ, Farrell J, et al. Sulfamethoxazole and its metabolite nitroso sulfamethoxazole stimulate dendritic cell costimulatory signaling. *J Immunol* 2007;178(9):5533-42.

[48] Chung WH, Hung SI, Yang JY, et al. Granulysin is a key mediator for disseminated keratinocyte death in Stevens-Johnson syndrome and toxic epidermal necrolysis. *Nat Med* 2008;14(12):1343-50.

[49] Gamen S, Hanson DA, Kaspar A, Naval J, Krensky AM, Anel A. Granulysin-induced apoptosis. I. Involvement of at least two distinct pathways. *J Immunol* 1998;161(4): 1758-64.

[50] Deng A, Chen S, Li Q, Lyu SC, Clayberger C, Krensky AM. Granulysin, a cytolytic molecule, is also a chemoattractant and proinflammatory activator. *J Immunol* 2005;174(9):5243-8.

[51] Viard I, Wehrli P, Bullani R, et al. Inhibition of toxic epidermal necrolysis by blockade of CD95 with human intravenous immunoglobulin. *Science* 1998;282(5388):490-3.

[52] Viard-Leveugle I, Bullani RR, Meda P, et al. Intracellular localization of keratinocyte Fas ligand explains lack of cytolytic activity under physiological conditions. *J Biol Chem* 2003;278(18):16183-8.

[53] Abe R, Shimizu T, Shibaki A, Nakamura H, Watanabe H, Shimizu H. Toxic epidermal necrolysis and Stevens-Johnson syndrome are induced by soluble Fas ligand. *Am J Pathol* 2003;162(5):1515-20.

[54] Nassif A, Bensussan A, Dorothee G, et al. Drug specific cytotoxic T-cells in the skin lesions of a patient with toxic epidermal necrolysis. *J Invest Dermatol* 2002;118(4): 728-33.

[55] Takahashi R, Kano Y, Yamazaki Y, Kimishima M, Mizukawa Y, Shiohara T. Defective regulatory T cells in patients with severe drug eruptions: timing of the dysfunction is associated with the pathological phenotype and outcome. *J Immunol* 2009;182(12): 8071-9.

[56] Posadas SJ, Padial A, Torres MJ, et al. Delayed reactions to drugs show levels of perforin, granzyme B, and Fas-L to be related to disease severity. *J Allergy Clin Immunol* 2002;109(1):155-61.

[57] Nassif A, Bensussan A, Boumsell L, et al. Toxic epidermal necrolysis: effector cells are drug-specific cytotoxic T cells. *J Allergy Clin Immunol* 2004;114(5):1209-15.

[58] Hung SI, Chung WH, Chen YT. HLA-B genotyping to detect carbamazepine induced Stevens-Johnson syndrome: implications for personalizing medicine. *Personalized Med.* 2005;2:225-237.

[59] Hung SI, Chung WH, Chen YT. Genetics of severe drug hypersensitivity reactions in Han Chinese. In: Pichler WJ, ed. Drug Hypersensitivity. Basel.: Karger., 2007: 105-114.

[60] Chung WH, Hung SI, Hong HS, et al. Medical genetics: a marker for Stevens-Johnson syndrome. *Nature* 2004;428(6982):486.

[61] Hung SI, Chung WH, Jee SH, et al. Genetic susceptibility to carbamazepine-induced cutaneous adverse drug reactions. *Pharmacogenet Genomics* 2006;16(4):297-306.

[62] Lonjou C, Thomas L, Borot N, et al. A marker for Stevens-Johnson syndrome ...: ethnicity matters. *Pharmacogenomics J* 2006;6(4):265-8.

[63] Kaniwa N, Saito Y, Aihara M, et al. HLA-B locus in Japanese patients with anti-epileptics and allopurinol-related Stevens-Johnson syndrome and toxic epidermal necrolysis. *Pharmacogenomics* 2008;9(11):1617-22.

[64] McCormack M, Alfirevic A, Bourgeois S, et al. HLA-A*3101 and carbamazepine-induced hypersensitivity reactions in Europeans. *N Engl J Med* 2011;364(12):1134-43.

[65] Ozeki T, Mushiroda T, Yowang A, et al. Genome-wide association study identifies HLA-A*3101 allele as a genetic risk factor for carbamazepine-induced cutaneous adverse drug reactions in Japanese population. *Hum Mol Genet* 2011;20(5):1034-41.

[66] Wen SH, Lai MJ, Yang KL. Human leukocyte antigen-A, -B, and -DRB1 haplotypes of cord blood units in the Tzu Chi Taiwan Cord Blood Bank. *Hum Immunol* 2008;69(7): 430-6.

[67] Hung SI, Chung WH, Liou LB, et al. HLA-B*5801 allele as a genetic marker for severe cutaneous adverse reactions caused by allopurinol. *Proc Natl Acad Sci U S A* 2005;102(11):4134-9.

[68] Lonjou C, Borot N, Sekula P, et al. A European study of HLA-B in Stevens-Johnson syndrome and toxic epidermal necrolysis related to five high-risk drugs. *Pharmacogenet Genomics* 2008;18(2):99-107.

[69] Daar AS, Singer PA. Pharmacogenetics and geographical ancestry: implications for drug development and global health. *Nat Rev Genet* 2005;6(3):241-6.

[70] Schmidt AH, Baier D, Solloch UV, et al. Estimation of high-resolution HLA-A, -B, -C, -DRB1 allele and haplotype frequencies based on 8862 German stem cell donors and implications for strategic donor registry planning. *Hum Immunol* 2009;70(11):895-902.

[71] Ueta M, Sotozono C, Inatomi T, Kojima K, Hamuro J, Kinoshita S. Association of Fas Ligand gene polymorphism with Stevens-Johnson syndrome. *Br J Ophthalmol* 2008;92(7):989-91.

[72] Ueta M, Sotozono C, Inatomi T, et al. Toll-like receptor 3 gene polymorphisms in Japanese patients with Stevens-Johnson syndrome. *Br J Ophthalmol* 2007;91(7):962-5.

[73] Ueta M, Sotozono C, Inatomi T, Kojima K, Hamuro J, Kinoshita S. Association of combined IL-13/IL-4R signaling pathway gene polymorphism with Stevens-Johnson syndrome accompanied by ocular surface complications. *Invest Ophthalmol Vis Sci* 2008;49(5):1809-13.

[74] http://formularyproductions.com/blackbox/carbamazepine.

[75] Chen P, Lin JJ, Lu CS, et al. Carbamazepine-induced toxic effects and HLA-B*1502 screening in Taiwan. *N Engl J Med* 2011;364(12):1126-33.

[76] Fernando SL, Broadfoot AJ. Prevention of severe cutaneous adverse drug reactions: the emerging value of pharmacogenetic screening. *Cmaj* 2010;182(5):476-80.

[77] Rauch A, Nolan D, Martin A, McKinnon E, Almeida C, Mallal S. Prospective genetic screening decreases the incidence of abacavir hypersensitivity reactions in the Western Australian HIV cohort study. *Clin Infect Dis* 2006;43(1):99-102.

[78] Halevy S, Ghislain PD, Mockenhaupt M, et al. Allopurinol is the most common cause of Stevens-Johnson syndrome and toxic epidermal necrolysis in Europe and Israel. *J Am Acad Dermatol* 2008;58(1):25-32.

[79] Stamp L, Gow P, Sharples K, Raill B. The optimal use of allopurinol: an audit of allopurinol use in South Auckland. *Aust N Z J Med* 2000;30(5):567-72.

[80] McInnes GT, Lawson DH, Jick H. Acute adverse reactions attributed to allopurinol in hospitalised patients. *Ann Rheum Dis* 1981;40(3):245-9.

[81] Hande KR, Noone RM, Stone WJ. Severe allopurinol toxicity. Description and guidelines for prevention in patients with renal insufficiency. *Am J Med* 1984;76(1):47-56.

[82] Kumar A, Edward N, White MI, Johnston PW, Catto GR. Allopurinol, erythema multiforme, and renal insufficiency. *Bmj* 1996;312(7024):173-4.

[83] Vazquez-Mellado J, Morales EM, Pacheco-Tena C, Burgos-Vargas R. Relation between adverse events associated with allopurinol and renal function in patients with gout. *Ann Rheum Dis* 2001;60(10):981-3.

[84] Dincer HE, Dincer AP, Levinson DJ. Asymptomatic hyperuricemia: to treat or not to treat. *Cleve Clin J Med* 2002;69(8):594, 597, 600-2 passim.

[85] Singer JZ, Wallace SL. The allopurinol hypersensitivity syndrome. Unnecessary morbidity and mortality. *Arthritis Rheum* 1986;29(1):82-7.

[86] Bellamy N, Brooks PM, Emmerson BT, Gilbert JR, Campbell J, McCredie M. A survey of current prescribing practices of anti-inflammatory and urate-lowering drugs in gouty arthritis in New South Wales and Queensland. *Med J Aust* 1989;151(9):531-2 535-7.

[87] Khoo BP, Leow YH. A review of inpatients with adverse drug reactions to allopurinol. *Singapore Med J* 2000;41(4):156-60.

[88] Schlienger RG, Shapiro LE, Shear NH. Lamotrigine-induced severe cutaneous adverse reactions. *Epilepsia* 1998;39 Suppl 7:S22-6.

[89] Mockenhaupt M, Messenheimer J, Tennis P, Schlingmann J. Risk of Stevens-Johnson syndrome and toxic epidermal necrolysis in new users of antiepileptics. *Neurology* 2005;64(7):1134-8.

[90] Yalcin B, Karaduman A. Stevens-Johnson syndrome associated with concomitant use of lamotrigine and valproic acid. *J Am Acad Dermatol* 2000;43(5 Pt 2):898-9.

[91] Wolkenstein P, Carriere V, Charue D, et al. A slow acetylator genotype is a risk factor for sulphonamide-induced toxic epidermal necrolysis and Stevens-Johnson syndrome. *Pharmacogenetics* 1995;5(4):255-8.

[92] Dietrich A, Kawakubo Y, Rzany B, Mockenhaupt M, Simon JC, Schopf E. Low N-acetylating capacity in patients with Stevens-Johnson syndrome and toxic epidermal necrolysis. *Exp Dermatol* 1995;4(5):313-6.

[93] Becker DS. Toxic epidermal necrolysis. *Lancet* 1998;351(9113):1417-20.

[94] Quinn AM, Brown K, Bonish BK, et al. Uncovering histologic criteria with prognostic significance in toxic epidermal necrolysis. *Arch Dermatol* 2005;141(6):683-7.

[95] Abe R, Yoshioka N, Murata J, Fujita Y, Shimizu H. Granulysin as a marker for early diagnosis of the Stevens-Johnson syndrome. *Ann Intern Med* 2009;151(7):514-5.

[96] Wolkenstein P, Chosidow O, Flechet ML, et al. Patch testing in severe cutaneous adverse drug reactions, including Stevens-Johnson syndrome and toxic epidermal necrolysis. *Contact Dermatitis* 1996;35(4):234-6.

[97] Kano Y, Hirahara K, Mitsuyama Y, Takahashi R, Shiohara T. Utility of the lymphocyte transformation test in the diagnosis of drug sensitivity: dependence on its timing and the type of drug eruption. *Allergy* 2007;62(12):1439-44.

[98] Zawodniak A, Lochmatter P, Yerly D, et al. In vitro detection of cytotoxic T and NK cells in peripheral blood of patients with various drug-induced skin diseases. *Allergy* 2010;65(3):376-84.

[99] Bronnimann M, Yawalkar N. Histopathology of drug-induced exanthems: is there a role in diagnosis of drug allergy? *Curr Opin Allergy Clin Immunol* 2005;5(4):317-21.

[100] Mockenhaupt M. Severe drug-induced skin reactions: clinical pattern, diagnostics and therapy. *J Dtsch Dermatol Ges* 2009;7(2):142-60; quiz 161-2.

[101] Mockenhaupt M, Idzko M, Grosber M, Schopf E, Norgauer J. Epidemiology of staphylococcal scalded skin syndrome in Germany. *J Invest Dermatol* 2005;124(4):700-3.

[102] Yamasaki O, Yamaguchi T, Sugai M, et al. Clinical manifestations of staphylococcal scalded-skin syndrome depend on serotypes of exfoliative toxins. *J Clin Microbiol* 2005;43(4):1890-3.

[103] Ladhani S. Recent developments in staphylococcal scalded skin syndrome. *Clin Microbiol Infect* 2001;7(6):301-7.

[104] Lappin E, Ferguson AJ. Gram-positive toxic shock syndromes. *Lancet Infect Dis* 2009;9(5):281-90.

[105] Tonev S, Vasileva S, Kadurina M. Depot sulfonamid associated linear IgA bullous dermatosis with erythema multiforme-like clinical features. *J Eur Acad Dermatol Venereol* 1998;11(2):165-8.

[106] Anhalt GJ, Kim SC, Stanley JR, et al. Paraneoplastic pemphigus. An autoimmune mucocutaneous disease associated with neoplasia. *N Engl J Med* 1990;323(25):1729-35.

[107] Wade MS, Black MM. Paraneoplastic pemphigus: a brief update. *Australas J Dermatol* 2005;46(1):1-8; quiz 9-10.

[108] Ayoub N. [Pemphigus and pemphigus-triggering drugs]. *Ann Dermatol Venereol* 2005;132(6-7 Pt 1):595.

[109] Brenner S, Bialy-Golan A, Ruocco V. Drug-induced pemphigus. *Clin Dermatol* 1998;16(3):393-7.

[110] Mutasim DF, Pelc NJ, Anhalt GJ. Drug-induced pemphigus. *Dermatol Clin* 1993;11(3): 463-71.

[111] Bastuji-Garin S, Joly P, Picard-Dahan C, et al. Drugs associated with bullous pemphigoid. A case-control study. *Arch Dermatol* 1996;132(3):272-6.

[112] Fellner MJ. Drug-induced bullous pemphigoid. *Clin Dermatol* 1993;11(4):515-20.

[113] Olasz EB, Yancey KB. Bullous pemphigoid and related subepidermal autoimmune blistering diseases. *Curr Dir Autoimmun* 2008;10:141-66.

[114] Correia O, Delgado L, Barbosa IL, Campilho F, Fleming-Torrinha J. Increased interleukin 10, tumor necrosis factor alpha, and interleukin 6 levels in blister fluid of toxic epidermal necrolysis. *J Am Acad Dermatol* 2002;47(1):58-62.

[115] Schulz JT, 3rd, Sheridan RL. Severe desquamating disorder after liver transplant: toxic epidermal necrolysis or graft versus host disease? *J Burns Wounds* 2006;5:e1.

[116] Vargas-Diez E, Garcia-Diez A, Marin A, Fernandez-Herrera J. Life-threatening graft-vs-host disease. *Clin Dermatol* 2005;23(3):285-300.

[117] Friedman KJ, LeBoit PE, Farmer ER. Acute follicular graft-vs-host reaction. A distinct clinicopathologic presentation. *Arch Dermatol* 1988;124(5):688-91.

[118] Lin JH, Sheu HM, Lee JY. Acute generalized exanthematous pustulosis with erythema multiforme-like lesions. *Eur J Dermatol* 2002;12(5):475-8.

[119] Garcia-Doval I, LeCleach L, Bocquet H, Otero XL, Roujeau JC. Toxic epidermal necrolysis and Stevens-Johnson syndrome: does early withdrawal of causative drugs decrease the risk of death? *Arch Dermatol* 2000;136(3):323-7.

[120] Palmieri TL, Greenhalgh DG, Saffle JR, et al. A multicenter review of toxic epidermal necrolysis treated in U.S. burn centers at the end of the twentieth century. *J Burn Care Rehabil* 2002;23(2):87-96.

[121] Schulz JT, Sheridan RL, Ryan CM, MacKool B, Tompkins RG. A 10-year experience with toxic epidermal necrolysis. *J Burn Care Rehabil* 2000;21(3):199-204.

[122] Shiga S, Cartotto R. What are the fluid requirements in toxic epidermal necrolysis? *J Burn Care Res* 2010;31(1):100-4.

[123] Mayes T, Gottschlich M, Khoury J, Warner P, Kagan R. Energy requirements of pediatric patients with Stevens-Johnson syndrome and toxic epidermal necrolysis. *Nutr Clin Pract* 2008;23(5):547-50.

[124] Gravante G, Esposito G, Piazzolla M, Marianetti M, Delogu D, Montone A. Nutrition of toxic epidermal necrolysis. *J Hum Nutr Diet* 2006;19(2):152-3; author reply 153-5.

[125] Spies M, Sanford AP, Aili Low JF, Wolf SE, Herndon DN. Treatment of extensive toxic epidermal necrolysis in children. *Pediatrics* 2001;108(5):1162-8.

[126] Dorafshar AH, Dickie SR, Cohn AB, et al. Antishear therapy for toxic epidermal necrolysis: an alternative treatment approach. *Plast Reconstr Surg* 2008;122(1):154-60.

[127] Dalli RL, Kumar R, Kennedy P, Maitz P, Lee S, Johnson R. Toxic epidermal necrolysis/Stevens-Johnson syndrome: current trends in management. *ANZ J Surg* 2007;77(8):671-6.

[128] Huang SH, Yang PS, Wu SH, et al. Aquacel Ag with Vaseline gauze in the management of toxic epidermal necrolysis (TEN). *Burns* 2009;36(1):121-6.

[129] Boorboor P, Vogt PM, Bechara FG, et al. Toxic epidermal necrolysis: use of Biobrane or skin coverage reduces pain, improves mobilisation and decreases infection in elderly patients. *Burns* 2008;34(4):487-92.

[130] Pruitt BA, Jr. Burn treatment for the unburned. *Jama* 1987;257(16):2207-8.

[131] Gomes JA, Romano A, Santos MS, Dua HS. Amniotic membrane use in ophthalmology. *Curr Opin Ophthalmol* 2005;16(4):233-40.

[132] Rasmussen JE. Erythema multiforme in children. Response to treatment with systemic corticosteroids. *Br J Dermatol* 1976;95(2):181-6.

[133] Engelhardt SL, Schurr MJ, Helgerson RB. Toxic epidermal necrolysis: an analysis of referral patterns and steroid usage. *J Burn Care Rehabil* 1997;18(6):520-4.

[134] Ginsburg CM. Stevens-Johnson syndrome in children. *Pediatr Infect Dis* 1982;1(3): 155-8.

[135] Halebian PH, Corder VJ, Madden MR, Finklestein JL, Shires GT. Improved burn center survival of patients with toxic epidermal necrolysis managed without corticosteroids. *Ann Surg* 1986;204(5):503-12.

[136] Guibal F, Bastuji-Garin S, Chosidow O, Saiag P, Revuz J, Roujeau JC. Characteristics of toxic epidermal necrolysis in patients undergoing long-term glucocorticoid therapy. *Arch Dermatol* 1995;131(6):669-72.

[137] Samimi SS, Siegfried E. Stevens-Johnson syndrome developing in a girl with systemic lupus erythematosus on high-dose corticosteroid therapy. *Pediatr Dermatol* 2002;19(1):52-5.

[138] Kakourou T, Klontza D, Soteropoulou F, Kattamis C. Corticosteroid treatment of erythema multiforme major (Stevens-Johnson syndrome) in children. *Eur J Pediatr* 1997;156(2):90-3.

[139] Criton S, Devi K, Sridevi PK, Asokan PU. Toxic epidermal necrolysis--a retrospective study. *Int J Dermatol* 1997;36(12):923-5.

[140] Kardaun SH, Jonkman MF. Dexamethasone pulse therapy for Stevens-Johnson syndrome/toxic epidermal necrolysis. *Acta Derm Venereol* 2007;87(2):144-8.

[141] Yamane Y, Aihara M, Tatewaki S, et al. [Analysis of treatments and deceased cases of severe adverse drug reactions--analysis of 46 cases of Stevens-Johnson syndrome and toxic epidermal necrolysis]. *Arerugi* 2009;58(5):537-47.

[142] Araki Y, Sotozono C, Inatomi T, et al. Successful treatment of Stevens-Johnson syndrome with steroid pulse therapy at disease onset. *Am J Ophthalmol* 2009;147(6): 1004-11, 1011 e1.

[143] Prins C, Vittorio C, Padilla RS, et al. Effect of high-dose intravenous immunoglobulin therapy in Stevens-Johnson syndrome: a retrospective, multicenter study. *Dermatology* 2003;207(1):96-9.

[144] Campione E, Marulli GC, Carrozzo AM, Chimenti MS, Costanzo A, Bianchi L. High-dose intravenous immunoglobulin for severe drug reactions: efficacy in toxic epidermal necrolysis. *Acta Derm Venereol* 2003;83(6):430-2.

[145] Metry DW, Jung P, Levy ML. Use of intravenous immunoglobulin in children with stevens-johnson syndrome and toxic epidermal necrolysis: seven cases and review of the literature. *Pediatrics* 2003;112(6 Pt 1):1430-6.

[146] Yang Y, Xu J, Li F, Zhu X. Combination therapy of intravenous immunoglobulin and corticosteroid in the treatment of toxic epidermal necrolysis and Stevens-Johnson syndrome: a retrospective comparative study in China. *Int J Dermatol* 2009;48(10): 1122-8.

[147] Bachot N, Revuz J, Roujeau JC. Intravenous immunoglobulin treatment for Stevens-Johnson syndrome and toxic epidermal necrolysis: a prospective noncomparative study showing no benefit on mortality or progression. *Arch Dermatol* 2003;139(1): 33-6.

[148] Brown KM, Silver GM, Halerz M, Walaszek P, Sandroni A, Gamelli RL. Toxic epidermal necrolysis: does immunoglobulin make a difference? *J Burn Care Rehabil* 2004;25(1):81-8.

[149] Shortt R, Gomez M, Mittman N, Cartotto R. Intravenous immunoglobulin does not improve outcome in toxic epidermal necrolysis. *J Burn Care Rehabil* 2004;25(3):246-55.

[150] Pasic S. Intravenous immunoglobulin in toxic epidermal necrolysis. *Int J Dermatol* 2006;45(9):1117-8.

[151] Schneck J, Fagot JP, Sekula P, Sassolas B, Roujeau JC, Mockenhaupt M. Effects of treatments on the mortality of Stevens-Johnson syndrome and toxic epidermal necrolysis: A retrospective study on patients included in the prospective EuroSCAR Study. *J Am Acad Dermatol* 2008;58(1):33-40.

[152] Renfro L, Grant-Kels JM, Daman LA. Drug-induced toxic epidermal necrolysis treated with cyclosporin. *Int J Dermatol* 1989;28(7):441-4.

[153] Zaki I, Patel S, Reed R, Dalziel KL. Toxic epidermal necrolysis associated with severe hypocalcaemia, and treated with cyclosporin. *Br J Dermatol* 1995;133(2):337-8.

[154] Sullivan JR, Watson A. Lamotrigine-induced toxic epidermal necrolysis treated with intravenous cyclosporin: a discussion of pathogenesis and immunosuppressive management. *Australas J Dermatol* 1996;37(4):208-12.

[155] Hewitt J, Ormerod AD. Toxic epidermal necrolysis treated with cyclosporin. *Clin Exp Dermatol* 1992;17(4):264-5.

[156] Jarrett P, Ha T, Snow J. Toxic epidermal necrolysis and cyclosporin. *Clin Exp Dermatol* 1997;22(5):254.

[157] Arevalo JM, Lorente JA, Gonzalez-Herrada C, Jimenez-Reyes J. Treatment of toxic epidermal necrolysis with cyclosporin A. *J Trauma* 2000;48(3):473-8.

[158] Robak E, Robak T, Gora-Tybor J, et al. Toxic epidermal necrolysis in a patient with severe aplastic anemia treated with cyclosporin A and G-CSF. *J Med* 2001;32(1-2): 31-9.

[159] Yung A, Agnew K, Snow J, Oliver F. Two unusual cases of toxic epidermal necrolysis. *Australas J Dermatol* 2002;43(1):35-8.

[160] Hashim N, Bandara D, Tan E, Ilchyshyn A. Early cyclosporine treatment of incipient toxic epidermal necrolysis induced by concomitant use of lamotrigine and sodium valproate. *Acta Derm Venereol* 2004;84(1):90-1.

[161] Valeyrie-Allanore L, Wolkenstein P, Brochard L, et al. Open trial of ciclosporin treatment for Stevens-Johnson syndrome and toxic epidermal necrolysis. *Br J Dermatol* 2010;163(4):847-53.

[162] Sakellariou G, Koukoudis P, Karpouzas J, et al. Plasma exchange (PE) treatment in drug-induced toxic epidermal necrolysis (TEN). *Int J Artif Organs* 1991;14(10):634-8.

[163] Chaidemenos GC, Chrysomallis F, Sombolos K, Mourellou O, Ioannides D, Papakonstantinou M. Plasmapheresis in toxic epidermal necrolysis. *Int J Dermatol* 1997;36(3): 218-21.

[164] Egan CA, Grant WJ, Morris SE, Saffle JR, Zone JJ. Plasmapheresis as an adjunct treatment in toxic epidermal necrolysis. *J Am Acad Dermatol* 1999;40(3):458-61.

[165] Bamichas G, Natse T, Christidou F, et al. Plasma exchange in patients with toxic epidermal necrolysis. *Ther Apher* 2002;6(3):225-8.

[166] Furubacke A, Berlin G, Anderson C, Sjoberg F. Lack of significant treatment effect of plasma exchange in the treatment of drug-induced toxic epidermal necrolysis? *Intensive Care Med* 1999;25(11):1307-10.

[167] Paquet P, Paquet F, Al Saleh W, Reper P, Vanderkelen A, Pierard GE. Immunoregulatory effector cells in drug-induced toxic epidermal necrolysis. *Am J Dermatopathol* 2000;22(5):413-7.

[168] Fischer M, Fiedler E, Marsch WC, Wohlrab J. Antitumour necrosis factor-alpha antibodies (infliximab) in the treatment of a patient with toxic epidermal necrolysis. *Br J Dermatol* 2002;146(4):707-9.

[169] Hunger RE, Hunziker T, Buettiker U, Braathen LR, Yawalkar N. Rapid resolution of toxic epidermal necrolysis with anti-TNF-alpha treatment. *J Allergy Clin Immunol* 2005;116(4):923-4.

[170] Meiss F, Helmbold P, Meykadeh N, Gaber G, Marsch W, Fischer M. Overlap of acute generalized exanthematous pustulosis and toxic epidermal necrolysis: response to antitumour necrosis factor-alpha antibody infliximab: report of three cases. *J Eur Acad Dermatol Venereol* 2007;21(5):717-9.

[171] Wojtkiewicz A, Wysocki M, Fortuna J, Chrupek M, Matczuk M, Koltan A. Beneficial and rapid effect of infliximab on the course of toxic epidermal necrolysis. *Acta Derm Venereol* 2008;88(4):420-1.

[172] Gubinelli E, Canzona F, Tonanzi T, Raskovic D, Didona B. Toxic epidermal necrolysis successfully treated with etanercept. *J Dermatol* 2009;36(3):150-3.

[173] Sadighha A. Etanercept in the treatment of a patient with acute generalized exanthematous pustulosis/toxic epidermal necrolysis: definition of a new model based on translational research. *Int J Dermatol* 2009;48(8):913-4.

[174] Velez A, Moreno JC. Toxic epidermal necrolysis treated with N-acetylcysteine. *J Am Acad Dermatol* 2002;46(3):469-70.

[175] Claes P, Wintzen M, Allard S, Simons P, De Coninck A, Lacor P. Nevirapine-induced toxic epidermal necrolysis and toxic hepatitis treated successfully with a combination of intravenous immunoglobulins and N-acetylcysteine. *Eur J Intern Med* 2004;15(4): 255-258.

[176] Paquet P, Jacob E, Damas P, Pierard GE. Recurrent fatal drug-induced toxic epidermal necrolysis (Lyell's syndrome) after putative beta-lactam cross-reactivity: Case report and scrutiny of antibiotic imputability. *Crit Care Med* 2002;30(11):2580-3.

[177] Lam A, Randhawa I, Klaustermeyer W. Cephalosporin induced toxic epidermal necrolysis and subsequent penicillin drug exanthem. *Allergol Int* 2008;57(3):281-4.

[178] Merritt HH, Putnam TJ. Sodium diphenylhydantoinate in the treatment of convulsive disorders. *JAMA* 1938;111:1068-1073.

[179] Chaiken BH, Goldberg BI, Segal JP. Dilantin sensitivity; report of a case of hepatitis with jaundice, pyrexia and exfoliative dermatitis. *N Engl J Med* 1950;242(23):897-8.

[180] Saltzstein SL, Ackerman LV. Lymphadenopathy induced by anticonvulsant drugs and mimicking clinically pathologically malignant lymphomas. *Cancer* 1959;12(1): 164-82.

[181] Shear NH, Spielberg SP. Anticonvulsant hypersensitivity syndrome. In vitro assessment of risk. *J Clin Invest* 1988;82(6):1826-32.

[182] Bocquet H, Bagot M, Roujeau JC. Drug-induced pseudolymphoma and drug hypersensitivity syndrome (Drug Rash with Eosinophilia and Systemic Symptoms: DRESS). *Semin Cutan Med Surg* 1996;15(4):250-7.

[183] Suzuki Y, Inagi R, Aono T, Yamanishi K, Shiohara T. Human herpesvirus 6 infection as a risk factor for the development of severe drug-induced hypersensitivity syndrome. *Arch Dermatol* 1998;134(9):1108-12.

[184] Shiohara T, Inaoka M, Kano Y. Drug-induced hypersensitivity syndrome (DIHS): a reaction induced by a complex interplay among herpesviruses and antiviral and antidrug immune responses. *Allergol Int* 2006;55(1):1-8.

[185] Gennis MA, Vemuri R, Burns EA, Hill JV, Miller MA, Spielberg SP. Familial occurrence of hypersensitivity to phenytoin. *Am J Med* 1991;91(6):631-4.

[186] Mockenhaupt M. Epidemiology and causes of severe cutaneous adverse drug reactions. In: Pichler WJ, ed. Drug hypersensitivity. Basel: Karger, 2007: 18-31.

[187] Kardaun SH, Sidoroff A, Valeyrie-Allanore L, et al. Variability in the clinical pattern of cutaneous side-effects of drugs with systemic symptoms: does a DRESS syndrome really exist? *Br J Dermatol* 2007;156(3):609-11.

[188] Shiohara T, Iijima M, Ikezawa Z, Hashimoto K. The diagnosis of a DRESS syndrome has been sufficiently established on the basis of typical clinical features and viral reactivations. *Br J Dermatol* 2007;156(5):1083-4.

[189] Kano Y, Inaoka M, Shiohara T. Association between anticonvulsant hypersensitivity syndrome and human herpesvirus 6 reactivation and hypogammaglobulinemia. *Arch Dermatol* 2004;140(2):183-8.

[190] Shiohara T, Takahashi R, Kano Y. Drug-induced hypersensitivity syndrome (DIHS): a reaction induced by a complex interplay among herpesviruses and antiviral and antidrug immune responses. In: Pichler WJ, ed. Allergol Int. Basel: Karger, 2007: 251-266.

[191] Roujeau JC, Stern RS. Severe adverse cutaneous reactions to drugs. *N Engl J Med* 1994;331(19):1272-85.

[192] Kano Y, Shiohara T. The variable clinical picture of drug-induced hypersensitivity syndrome/drug rash with eosinophilia and systemic symptoms in relation to the eliciting drug. *Immunol Allergy Clin North Am* 2009;29(3):481-501.

[193] Mallal S, Nolan D, Witt C, et al. Association between presence of HLA-B*5701, HLA-DR7, and HLA-DQ3 and hypersensitivity to HIV-1 reverse-transcriptase inhibitor abacavir. *Lancet* 2002;359(9308):727-32.

[194] Ben m'rad M, Leclerc-Mercier S, Blanche P, et al. Drug-induced hypersensitivity syndrome: clinical and biologic disease patterns in 24 patients. *Medicine (Baltimore)* 2009;88(3):131-40.

[195] Masaki T, Fukunaga A, Tohyama M, et al. Human herpes virus 6 encephalitis in allopurinol-induced hypersensitivity syndrome. *Acta Derm Venereol* 2003;83(2):128-31.

[196] Sakuma K, Kano Y, Fukuhara M, Shiohara T. Syndrome of inappropriate secretion of antidiuretic hormone associated with limbic encephalitis in a patient with drug-induced hypersensitivity syndrome. *Clin Exp Dermatol* 2008;33(3):287-90.

[197] Asano Y, Kagawa H, Kano Y, Shiohara T. Cytomegalovirus disease during severe drug eruptions: report of 2 cases and retrospective study of 18 patients with drug-induced hypersensitivity syndrome. *Arch Dermatol* 2009;145(9):1030-6.

[198] Descamps V, Bouscarat F, Laglenne S, et al. Human herpesvirus 6 infection associated with anticonvulsant hypersensitivity syndrome and reactive haemophagocytic syndrome. *Br J Dermatol* 1997;137(4):605-8.

[199] Lazoglu AH, Boglioli LR, Dorsett B, Macris NT. Phenytoin-related immunodeficiency associated with Loeffler's syndrome. *Ann Allergy Asthma Immunol* 1995;74(6): 479-82.

[200] Kano Y, Hiraharas K, Sakuma K, Shiohara T. Several herpesviruses can reactivate in a severe drug-induced multiorgan reaction in the same sequential order as in graft-versus-host disease. *Br J Dermatol* 2006;155(2):301-6.

[201] Aota N, Shiohara T. Viral connection between drug rashes and autoimmune diseases: how autoimmune responses are generated after resolution of drug rashes. *Autoimmun Rev* 2009;8(6):488-94.

[202] Chiou CC, Chung WH, Hung SI, Yang LC, Hong HS. Fulminant type 1 diabetes mellitus caused by drug hypersensitivity syndrome with human herpesvirus 6 infection. *J Am Acad Dermatol* 2006;54(2 Suppl):S14-7.

[203] Ozaki N, Miura Y, Sakakibara A, Oiso Y. A case of hypersensitivity syndrome induced by methimazole for Graves' disease. *Thyroid* 2005;15(12):1333-6.

[204] Kano Y, Sakuma K, Shiohara T. Sclerodermoid graft-versus-host disease-like lesions occurring after drug-induced hypersensitivity syndrome. *Br J Dermatol* 2007;156(5): 1061-3.

[205] Aota N, Hirahara K, Kano Y, Fukuoka T, Yamada A, Shiohara T. Systemic lupus erythematosus presenting with Kikuchi-Fujimoto's disease as a long-term sequela of

drug-induced hypersensitivity syndrome. A possible role of Epstein-Barr virus reactivation. *Dermatology* 2009;218(3):275-7.

[206] Kijima A, Inui S, Nakamura T, Itami S, Katayama I. Does drug-induced hypersensitivity syndrome elicit bullous pemphigoid? *Allergol Int* 2008;57(2):181-2.

[207] Hetherington S, McGuirk S, Powell G, et al. Hypersensitivity reactions during therapy with the nucleoside reverse transcriptase inhibitor abacavir. *Clin Ther* 2001;23(10): 1603-14.

[208] Peyriere H, Guillemin V, Lotthe A, et al. Reasons for early abacavir discontinuation in HIV-infected patients. *Ann Pharmacother* 2003;37(10):1392-7.

[209] Peyriere H, Dereure O, Breton H, et al. Variability in the clinical pattern of cutaneous side-effects of drugs with systemic symptoms: does a DRESS syndrome really exist? *Br J Dermatol* 2006;155(2):422-8.

[210] Fernando SL, Henderson CJ, O'Connor KS. Drug-induced hypersensitivity syndrome with superficial granulomatous dermatitis--a novel finding. *Am J Dermatopathol* 2009;31(6):611-3.

[211] Santiago F, Goncalo M, Vieira R, Coelho S, Figueiredo A. Epicutaneous patch testing in drug hypersensitivity syndrome (DRESS). *Contact Dermatitis* 2010;62(1):47-53.

[212] Phillips EJ, Wong GA, Kaul R, et al. Clinical and immunogenetic correlates of abacavir hypersensitivity. *Aids* 2005;19(9):979-81.

[213] Hirahara K, Kano Y, Mitsuyama Y, Takahashi R, Kimishima M, Shiohara T. Differences in immunological alterations and underlying viral infections in two well-defined severe drug eruptions. *Clin Exp Dermatol* 2010;35(8):863-8.

[214] Hughes AR, Mosteller M, Bansal AT, et al. Association of genetic variations in HLA-B region with hypersensitivity to abacavir in some, but not all, populations. *Pharmacogenomics* 2004;5(2):203-11.

[215] Park WB, Choe PG, Song KH, et al. Should HLA-B*5701 screening be performed in every ethnic group before starting abacavir? *Clin Infect Dis* 2009;48(3):365-7.

[216] Cao K, Hollenbach J, Shi X, Shi W, Chopek M, Fernandez-Vina MA. Analysis of the frequencies of HLA-A, B, and C alleles and haplotypes in the five major ethnic groups of the United States reveals high levels of diversity in these loci and contrasting distribution patterns in these populations. *Hum Immunol* 2001;62(9):1009-30.

[217] Mallal S, Phillips E, Carosi G, et al. HLA-B*5701 screening for hypersensitivity to abacavir. *N Engl J Med* 2008;358(6):568-79.

[218] Fields KS, Petersen MJ, Chiao E, Tristani-Firouzi P. Case reports: treatment of nevirapine-associated dress syndrome with intravenous immune globulin (IVIG). *J Drugs Dermatol* 2005;4(4):510-3.

[219] Santos RP, Ramilo O, Barton T. Nevirapine-associated rash with eosinophilia and systemic symptoms in a child with human immunodeficiency virus infection. *Pediatr Infect Dis J* 2007;26(11):1053-6.

[220] Higuchi M, Agatsuma T, Iizima M, et al. A case of drug-induced hypersensitivity syndrome with multiple organ involvement treated with plasma exchange. *Ther Apher Dial* 2005;9(5):412-6.

[221] Shaughnessy KK, Bouchard SM, Mohr MR, Herre JM, Salkey KS. Minocycline-induced drug reaction with eosinophilia and systemic symptoms (DRESS) syndrome with persistent myocarditis. *J Am Acad Dermatol* 2010;62(2):315-8.

[222] Beylot C, Bioulac P, Doutre MS. [Acute generalized exanthematic pustuloses (four cases) (author's transl)]. *Ann Dermatol Venereol* 1980;107(1-2):37-48.

[223] Sidoroff A, Halevy S, Bavinck JN, Vaillant L, Roujeau JC. Acute generalized exanthematous pustulosis (AGEP)--a clinical reaction pattern. *J Cutan Pathol* 2001;28(3): 113-9.

[224] Chang SL, Huang YH, Yang CH, Hu S, Hong HS. Clinical manifestations and characteristics of patients with acute generalized exanthematous pustulosis in Asia. *Acta Derm Venereol* 2008;88(4):363-5.

[225] Davidovici B, Dodiuk-Gad R, Rozenman D, Halevy S. Profile of acute generalized exanthematous pustulosis in Israel during 2002-2005: results of the RegiSCAR Study. *Isr Med Assoc J* 2008;10(6):410-2.

[226] Zhang JL, Chen X, Li J, Xie HF. [Clinical analysis of childhood acute generalized exanthematous pustulosis]. *Zhongguo Dang Dai Er Ke Za Zhi* 2008;10(4):497-9.

[227] Roujeau JC. Clinical heterogeneity of drug hypersensitivity. *Toxicology* 2005;209(2): 123-9.

[228] Brandenburg VM, Kurts C, Eitner F, Hamilton-Williams E, Heintz B. Acute reversible renal failure in acute generalized exanthematous pustulosis. *Nephrol Dial Transplant* 2002;17(10):1857-8.

[229] Belhadjali H, Mandhouj S, Moussa A, et al. Mercury-induced acute generalized exanthematous pustulosis misdiagnosed as a drug-related case. *Contact Dermatitis* 2008;59(1):52-4.

[230] Belhadjali H, Ghannouchi N, Njim L, et al. Acute generalized exanthematous pustulosis induced by bufexamac in an atopic girl. *Contact Dermatitis* 2008;58(4):247-8.

[231] Rouchouse B, Bonnefoy M, Pallot B, Jacquelin L, Dimoux-Dime G, Claudy AL. Acute generalized exanthematous pustular dermatitis and viral infection. *Dermatologica* 1986;173(4):180-4.

[232] Feio AB, Apetato M, Costa MM, Sa J, Alcantara J. [Acute generalized exanthematous pustulosis due to Coxsackie B4 virus]. *Acta Med Port* 1997;10(6-7):487-91.

[233] Haro-Gabaldon V, Sanchez-Sanchez-Vizcaino J, Ruiz-Avila P, Gutierrez-Fernandez J, Linares J, Naranjo-Sintes R. Acute generalized exanthematous pustulosis with cytomegalovirus infection. *Int J Dermatol* 1996;35(10):735-7.

[234] Naides SJ. Rheumatic manifestations of parvovirus B19 infection. *Rheum Dis Clin North Am* 1998;24(2):375-401.

[235] Manzano S, Guggisberg D, Hammann C, Laubscher B. [Acute generalized exanthematous pustulosis: first case associated with a Chlamydia pneumoniae infection]. *Arch Pediatr* 2006;13(9):1230-2.

[236] Klein N, Hartmann M, Helmbold P, Enk A. [Acute generalized exanthematous pustulosis associated with recurrent urinary tract infections]. *Hautarzt* 2009;60(3):226-8.

[237] Davidovici BB, Pavel D, Cagnano E, Rozenman D, Halevy S. Acute generalized exanthematous pustulosis following a spider bite: report of 3 cases. *J Am Acad Dermatol* 2006;55(3):525-9.

[238] Birnie AJ, Litlewood SM. Acute generalized exanthematous pustulosis does not always have a drug-related cause. *Br J Dermatol* 2008;159(2):492-3.

[239] Schmid S, Kuechler PC, Britschgi M, et al. Acute generalized exanthematous pustulosis: role of cytotoxic T cells in pustule formation. *Am J Pathol* 2002;161(6):2079-86.

[240] Schaerli P, Britschgi M, Keller M, et al. Characterization of human T cells that regulate neutrophilic skin inflammation. *J Immunol* 2004;173(3):2151-8.

[241] Lazarov A, Livni E, Halevy S. Generalized pustular drug eruptions: confirmation by in vitro tests. *J Eur Acad Dermatol Venereol* 1998;10(1):36-41.

[242] Halevy S, Cohen A, Livni E. Acute generalized exanthematous pustulosis associated with polysensitivity to paracetamol and bromhexine: the diagnostic role of in vitro interferon-gamma release test. *Clin Exp Dermatol* 2000;25(8):652-4.

[243] Girardi M, Duncan KO, Tigelaar RE, Imaeda S, Watsky KL, McNiff JM. Cross-comparison of patch test and lymphocyte proliferation responses in patients with a history of acute generalized exanthematous pustulosis. *Am J Dermatopathol* 2005;27(4): 343-6.

[244] Britschgi M, Steiner UC, Schmid S, et al. T-cell involvement in drug-induced acute generalized exanthematous pustulosis. *J Clin Invest* 2001;107(11):1433-41.

[245] Mashiah J, Brenner S. A systemic reaction to patch testing for the evaluation of acute generalized exanthematous pustulosis. *Arch Dermatol* 2003;139(9):1181-3.

[246] Thomas E, Bellon T, Barranco P, et al. Acute generalized exanthematous pustulosis due to tetrazepam. *J Investig Allergol Clin Immunol* 2008;18(2):119-22.

[247] Halevy S, Cohen AD, Grossman N. Clinical implications of in vitro drug-induced interferon gamma release from peripheral blood lymphocytes in cutaneous adverse drug reactions. *J Am Acad Dermatol* 2005;52(2):254-61.

[248] Tamir E, Wohl Y, Mashiah J, Brenner S. Acute generalized exanthematous pustulosis: a retrospective analysis showing a clear predilection for women. *Skinmed* 2006;5(4): 186-8.

Chapter 5

Pemphigus Vulgaris and Pemphigus Foliaceus

Suran L. Fernando, Jamma Li and Mark Schifter

Additional information is available at the end of the chapter

http://dx.doi.org/10.5772/56423

1. Introduction

The word "pemphigus" is derived from the Greek term "pemphix" meaning bubble or blister. Pemphigus is a group of autoimmune diseases (see Table 4) characterized by intra-epithelial blistering, resulting in superficial vesicles or bullae that easily rupture, resulting in ulceration of mucosal and/or cutaneous sites. Although rare, pemphigus causes significant morbidity and potential mortality for patients. The two main subtypes are pemphigus vulgaris (PV), and pemphigus foliaceous (PF), of which PV is the most common and clinically, the most aggressive variant, being associated with significant morbidity and mortality, composing 70% of all reported cases of pemphigus: Less common forms and variants include paraneoplastic pemphigus, drug induced pemphigus, and IgA pemphigus. This book chapter focuses on the diagnosis and treatment of PV and PF.

2. Epidemiology

The estimated incidence of pemphigus is 1-16 cases per year per million people [1],[2]. PV is the most common type of pemphigus found in the USA and Europe. In the USA, PV is 5 times as prevalent as PF [3]. In contrast, PF is more common in certain countries such as Finland and South Africa [4] and the endemic variety, Fogo Salvegem, affects up to 3% of the population, in affected rural regions in Brazil, Columbia, and Tunisia [5]-[7].

3. Pathogenesis

The pathogenesis of pemphigus involves the targeting of inter-keratinocyte adhesion molecules by autoantibodies, leading to acantholysis and subsequent blister formation. There are four subtypes of desmoglein, which are glycoproteins that belong to a superfamily of cadherin molecules and are essential components of desmosomal intracellular adhesive junctions [8]. The molecular target in PF is desmoglein-1, which is found predominantly in the upper layers of the epidermis of the skin [9] [10]. Two subtypes of PV are described. In mucosal-dominant PV, the molecular target is restricted to desmoglein-3, whereas in mucocutaneous PV, the target is desmoglein-3 and desmoglein-1.[8] Desmoglein-3 is found in mucous membranes and predominantly in the lower layers of the epidermis of the skin and hence explains the absence of mucous membrane involvement in PF. Current evidence suggests that autoantibodies to desmogleins cause the loss of this desmosome from the surface of the keratinocyte and rearrangement of the actin cytoskeleton. This results in an unidentified cascade of signalling events resulting in apoptotic cell death and acantholysis [11]. Autoantibodies to desmoglein-3 and desmoglein-1 are paramount in the pathogenesis of PV and PF. In PV, this is demonstrated by the fact that passive transfer of serum IgG to desmoglein-3 into newborn mice induces blister formation [12].

Interaction between antigen specific T cells and B cells is postulated for the production of antibodies to desmoglein-3 and desmoglein-1. Autoantibody production has been shown, in vitro, to be dependent on mononuclear cells [13]. Further, aberrant T cell recognition of desmoglein-3 and desmoglein-1 is likely involved in the initiation and perpetuation of the B cell response.

Additionally, in PV, HLA Class 2 alleles including HLA DRβ1*0402, β1*1401, β1*0503 may be involved in the presentation of desmoglein-3 peptides to autoreactive T cells. However, similar associations are not observed in PF [14]. Further it has been observed that autoantibodies of the Th2-dependent IgG4 subtype are present in active disease but are not detectable in inactive disease or healthy individuals [15]. In active disease, IgG1 and IgG4 recognises epitopes in EC1 (amino acids 50-79, Bos 1) and EC2 (amino acids 200-29, Bos 2) of desmoglein-3. In inactive disease, only autoantibodies of the Th1-dependent IgG1 subtype to EC1 are detectable [15]. These observations suggest that IgG4 against EC2 is the main antibody responsible for acantholysis, but that this process may be facilitated or enhanced by IgG4 against EC1 [14].

A Th2 response predominates in PV. This suggests that Th2 cells are needed to activate B cells to initiate antibody production [16]. Further, in PV and PF, imbalance between Th2 and Th1 cytokines in terms of the elevation of the former against the suppression of the latter is postulated to contribute to pathogenesis [16],[17]. It is possible that Th17 and Treg pathways may also be integral. However, the association between Th cell subsets and disease activity is not well understood.

PV autoantibodies also bind large portions of keratinocytes outside desmosomal structures. Autoantibodies against other keratinocyte surface antigens such as desmoglein-4, desmocollins, acetylcholine receptors, pemphaxin and α-9 acetylcholine receptors, of which some or maybe all, may be involved in the pathogenesis of PV [8]. It is not clear whether blister formation is a direct result of these antibodies or occurs indirectly through immune mediated pathways which involve inflammatory cells and cytokines [14]. For instance, TNF-α is observed to be raised in PV compared to healthy controls, and may also increase with disease activity [16],[18].

http://dx.doi.org/10.5772/56423

Genetic susceptibility by individuals that increases their risk for developing pemphigus is suggested by studies describing associations between certain HLA polymorphisms and subtypes of disease. For instance, HLA-DRB*0102, 0404, 1402, and 1406 have been associated with endemic PF [5]. In 87 Italian patients, 61 with PV and 26 with PF, it was found that pemphigus vulgaris and pemphigus foliaceus share HLA-DRB1*1401 and DQB1*0503, are both associated with both PV and PF, whereas DRB1*0402 is only prevalent in patients with PV [19]. In a group of 20 French patients [20] the HLA alleles DRB1*0404 and DRB1*0102 were found to be associated with PF. It remains to be determined, whether these HLA-polymorphisms are true disease susceptibility genes given their role in antigen presentation. Alternatively, they may be markers of disease susceptibility through strong linkage disequilibrium with the causative gene. An environmental trigger may ultimately result in expression if disease in genetically susceptible individuals as is suspected to occur in endemic PF in Brazil[21]. Recently, it has been postulated that the inciting antigen in Brazil is a salivary protein from a haematophagous black fly, *Simulium nigrimanum* [22].

Disease and Subtype(s) ***(alternate terms)***		**Clinical Presentation**		**Natural History/ Prognosis/ Outcome**	**Target Antigens**
Oral	Cutaneous				
Pemphigus vulgaris (PV)		Common. Usually the first site involved	Commonest and most aggressive form of pemphigus: oral mucosal involvement common and often first site of presentation leading to extensive skin involvement.	Fatal if untreated Good with treatment	Desmoglein 3 (Dsg 3 is more common in oral epithelium) (& Desmoglein 1 (Dsg-1 & 3 are both found in skin))
	Pemphigus vegetans	Rare (in all 3 forms of pemphigus vegetans)	Uncommon and less aggressive clinical variant of PV: presents with large verrucous confluent plaques and pustules localized to flexural areas (axilla/groin).	Often progresses to pemphigus vulgaris	
	Pemphigus vegetans of Neumann		Often begins and ends as typical PV. Needs more intense immune-suppression than seen with PV, with patients troubled by chronic relapses (and remissions).	Frequent relapses (even with treatment)	
	Pemphigus vegetans of Hallopeau		Relatively benign, usually very well localised disease.	Prolonged remission (with treatment)	
Pemphigus foliaceus (PF)		Rare	All forms of PF are characterised clinically by superficial cutaneous blisters and erosions seen on histology as subcorneal acantholysis.	More benign course than PV, with prolonged remission.	Desmoglein 1
	Pemphigus erythematosus ("Senear-Usher syndrome")		Very rare condition with the combined features of pemphigus foliaceus and SLE		

Disease and Subtype(s) ***(alternate terms)***		**Clinical Presentation**	**Natural History/ Prognosis/ Outcome**	**Target Antigens**
Endemic pemphigus ("Brazillian pemphigus" or "Fogo Sevagem" (FS))	Common (endemic form)	PF and FS are identical clinically, histologically, and serologically but differ significantly, *epidemiologically*, with marked geographic clustering in Brazil, being a diseases of people resident in/or near the rainforests. The autoimmune response in FS is thought to be triggered by a putative environmental factor.		
IgA pemphigus	Rare (all 3 forms of IgA pemphigus)	Rare, characterised by pruritic, flaccid vesicles and/or pustules in annular pattern with central crusting, sometimes hypopyon* of the eye. Pathogenesis: related to the neutrophilic infiltrate in the epidermis rather than solely to the binding of IgA to target epidermal antigens. DIF: IgA (cf IgG seen in all other forms of pemphigus) deposits in lower epithelium or entire epidermal cell surfaces	Recalcitrant to treatment with corticosteroids	Desmoglein 3 (& Desmoglein 1)
Subcorneal pustular dermatosis *("Sneddon-Wilkinson disease")*		Subcorneal (beneath the stratum corneum) blister containing neutrophils with epidermal acanthosis and spongiosis, results in superficial fragile blistering.		
Intraepidermal neutrophilic IgA dermatosis		Deeper, intra-epidermal blister containing neutrophils with epidermal acanthosis and spongiosis, results in more marked blistering and consequent ulceration.		
Paraneoplastic pemphigus	Common & very severe	Polymorphous skin eruption, consisting of blisters, erosions, and targetoid lesions; severe mucous membrane involvement. DIF: IgG deposits on entire epidermal cell surfaces +/- granular-linear complement auto-antibodies to rat bladder epithelium in 75% of cases.	Fatal	Desmoglein 3, Desmoplakin 1, Desmoplakin 2, BP 230, evoplakin, periplakin, others
Familial benign chronic pemphigus *("Hailey-Hailey disease")*	Rare	Not a true form of pemphigus, as it is not antibody mediated. It presents a chronic recurrent bullous and vesicular dermatitis of intertriginous areas that is characterized histologically by suprabasilar acantholysis.	chronic, relapsing–remitting course	Desmocollin 1

http://dx.doi.org/10.5772/56423

Disease and Subtype(s) *(alternate terms)*	Clinical Presentation	Natural History/ Prognosis/ Outcome	Target Antigens
	Pathogenesis: heterozygous mutations of the ATP2C1 gene leads to a malfunction of the encoded protein hPMR1 - hPMR1 being a high-affinity calcium transport ATPase pump of the Golgi complex. A low level of intracellular Ca2+ induces premature keratinocyte proliferation, which leads to dysfunctional desmosomal proteins and thus abnormal keratinocyte adhesion.		

PV = pemphigus vulgaris; PF = pemphigus foliaceous, SLE = systemic lupus erythematosus, FS = Fogo Sevagem, DIF = direct immune-fluorescence,

cf = in contrast, BP = bullous pemphigoid, AD = autosomal dominant inheritance, Ca^{2+} = calcium ion

*hypopyon= sterile leukocytic exudate, seen in the anterior chamber of the eye

Table 1. Clinical and Immunohistochemical Variants of Pemphigus

4. Clinical features

4.1. Pemphigus vulgaris

Patients with PV usually present, in the initial stage, with highly painful erosions of the oral mucosa (Figures 1, 2) [23], but other mucous membranes such as the nasal, laryngo-esophageal, genital, anal and conjunctival mucosae can be involved. Some patients have mucosal dominant disease whereas in others cutaneous lesions develop and manifest as flaccid blisters followed by denuding and ulceration (Figure 3). A direct Nikolksy's sign can be elicited where tangential pressure on the on perilesional skin causes the epidermis to separate from the dermis. Skin lesions have a predilection for the trunk, groins, axillae, scalp, face, and pressure points. Secondary infection and dehydration are frequent cause of morbidity and mortality. Studies that differentiate PV according to clinical phenotype have shown a lower mortality in patients with predominantly mucosal PV (1–17%) compared with those with mucocutaneous PV (34–42%)[24].

4.2. Pemphigus foliaceus

Non-endemic PF usually presents in middle age or older adults whereas endemic PF is more common in children and young adults. FS in Tunisian affect women 4 times as often as men [7]. In both non-endemic and endemic PF, patients usually report the eruption of blisters on the scalp, face and upper trunk but they are fragile and some patients present instead with multiple painful crusted erosions (Figure 4). There is no history of mucosal involvement.

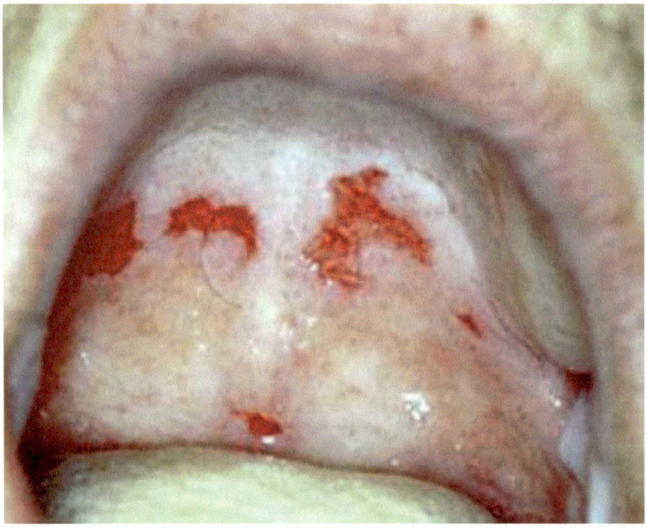

Figure 1. Pemphigus vulgaris with palatal ulceration and bleeding

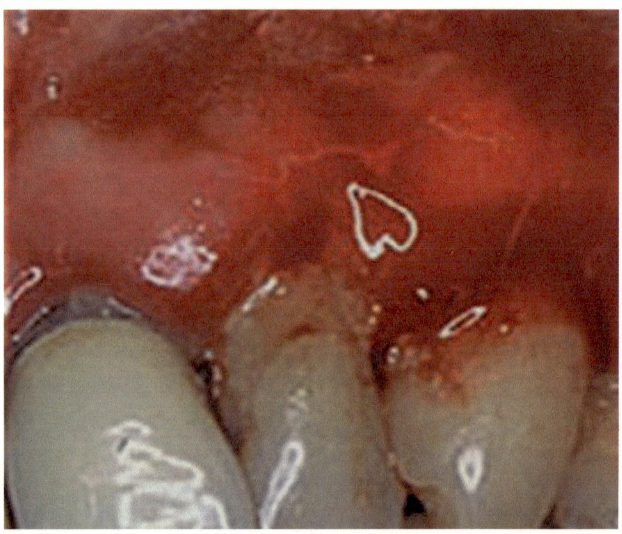

Figure 2. Pemphigus vulgaris with desquamative gingivitis

Pemphigus erythematosus is considered to be combination of PF and systemic lupus erythematosus typified by the presence of erosions in a malar distribution. Drug-associated cases may implicate angiotensin-converting enzyme inhibitors [25], penicillamine [26] or rifampicin [27]. There may be an intercurrent medical history of bullous pemphigoid [28], myasthenia gravis [29] or other autoimmune diseases [30]. PF has been associated with various malignancies such as non-Hodgkin's lymphoma [31], prostate cancer [32], and cutaneous squamous cell cancer [33].

http://dx.doi.org/10.5772/56423

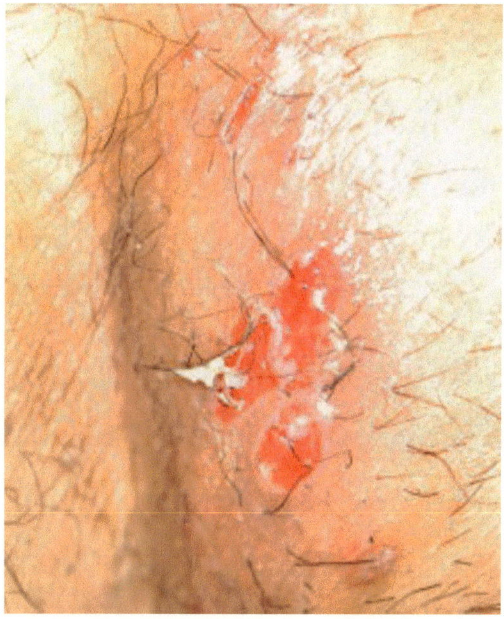

Figure 3. Pemphigus vulgaris characterised by multiple ulcers over the lower back

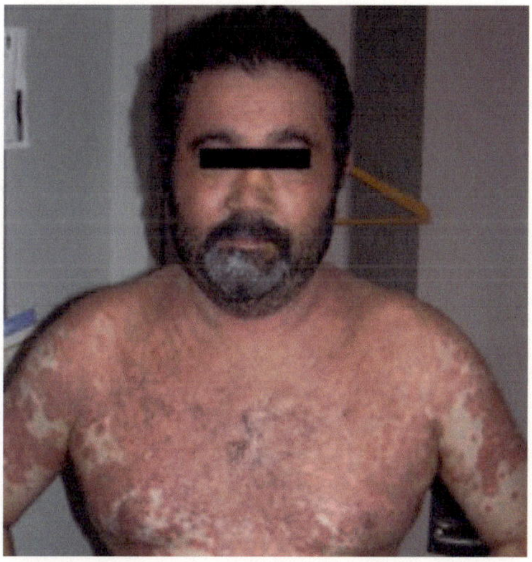

Figure 4. Pemphigus foliaceus characterised by exfoliative erythroderma

In both non-endemic and endemic PF, superficial flaccid vesicles and bullae may be evident and a positive Nikolsky sign is commonly elicited. However, the fragility of these lesions result in the formation of scaled erosions reflecting detachment of the stratum corneum from the stratum granulosum described as a 'corn flakes' appearance (Figure 5). At the severe end of the spectrum, PF can result in an exfoliative erythroderma.

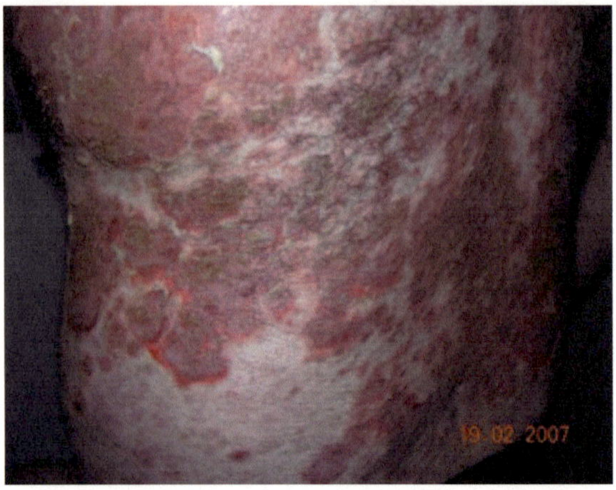

Figure 5. Pemphigus foliaceus with large scaly and crusted erosions over the trunk giving a 'corn flakes' appearance

PF causes significant morbidity as the lesions are painful and patients are prone to secondary infection, dehydration and metabolic disturbances with fatalities reported for those cases involving exfoliative erythroderma.

4.3. Differential diagnosis

Clinically, the differential diagnosis for mucosal lesions of PV (before the development of cutaneous disease) includes herpes simplex virus, lichen planus, mucous membrane (cicatricial) pemphigoid: erythema multiforme, and paraneoplastic pemphigus. The differential diagnosis for cutaneous involvement include other autoimmune blistering skin conditions, such as pemphigus foliaceus, pemphigus vegetans, IgA pemphigus, paraneoplastic pemphigus, bullous pemphigoid, linear IgA disease, erythema multiforme, Grover's disease, and Hailey-Hailey disease.

The differential diagnosis of endemic and nonendemic PF includes bullous impetigo, IgA pemphigus, pemphigus herpetiformis, drug eruptions, subcorneal pustular dermatosis, and systemic lupus erythematosus. If lesions are localized to the face or scalp with abundant scaling and yellow crusting, seborrheic dermatitis needs to be considered. The differential diagnosis of exfoliative erythroderma as the manifestation of PF includes papulosquamous diseases such as psoriasis, pityriasis rubra pilaris, and Drug Reaction with Eosinophilia and Systemic Symptoms.

5. Diagnosis

5.1. Histopathology

In PV, biopsy of lesional skin demonstrates intraepidermal splitting that occurs suprabasally forming an intraepidermal blister [34]. A single layer of basal keratinocytes remains attached

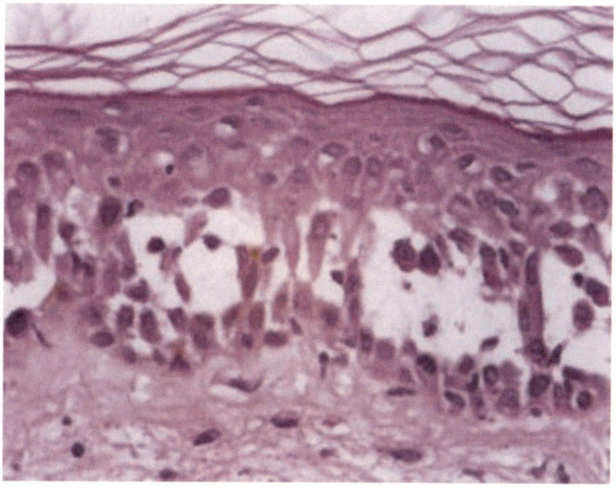

Figure 6. Medium power view of a skin biopsy from a patient with pemphigus vulgaris showing acantholysis of the suprabasal keratinocytes leaving a single layer of basal keratinocytes attached to the basement membrane (tombstone pattern), which forms the floor of an intraepidermal blister. The roof of the blister comprises relatively intact superficial epidermal layers with the stratum corneum. A sparse perivascular lymphocytic and eosinophilic inflammatory infiltrate is found within the upper dermis.

to the basement membrane (tombstone pattern), which forms the floor of the blister. The roof of the blister comprises relatively intact superficial epidermal layers with the stratum corneum showing a basketweave pattern. Hematoxylin and eosin staining demonstrates suprabasalar acantholysis and infiltration with predominantly neutrophils and eosinophils. A sparse perivascular lymphocytic and eosinophilic inflammatory infiltrate is found in the upper dermis [35] (Figure 6). In contrast, intraepidermal splitting is found subcorneally in PF with the initial formation of vacuoles within the intercellular spaces of the granular and/or upper spinous layers of the epidermis. [34] The vacuoles become larger and eventually lead to subcorneal blister formation within the upper epidermis (Figure 7). Hematoxylin and eosin staining show variable amounts of acantholytic keratinocytes, neutrophils, and fibrin within the blisters (Figure 8). Chronic PF lesions may show evidence of papillomatosis, acanthosis, hyperkeratosis, parakeratosis, and follicular plugging. The papillary dermis contains an inflammatory infiltrate composed of small numbers of neutrophils, eosinophils, and lymphocytes.

5.2. Direct immunofluorescence

Biopsy for direct immunofluorescence should be taken from perilesional mucosa and/orskin [36]. Biopsy of lesional tissue is not useful as immunoreactants are rapidly degraded by inflammatory activity [37]. To prevent the destruction of immunoreactants, specimens must be snap frozen and stored at temperatures below -70°C or placed in special transport media (such as Michel's medium) [36]. In direct immunofluorescence, specimens are incubated with fluorescein isothiocyanate-labelled antibodies against immunoglobulins, complement or fibrinogen, and examined with a fluorescent microscope [36]. In PV, direct immunofluores-

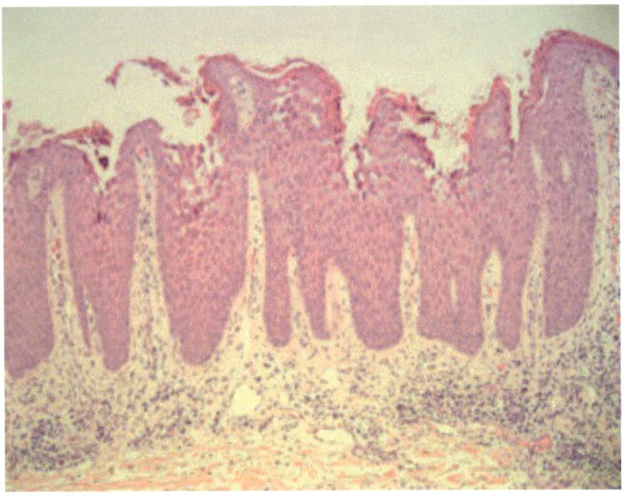

Figure 7. Medium power view of a skin biopsy from a patient with pemphigus foliaceus showing vacuoles within the intercellular spaces of the stratum granulosum and the upper stratum spinosum of the epidermis. The papillary dermis contains an inflammatory infiltrate comprising neutrophils, eosinophils, and lymphocytes (hematoxylin and eosin staining).

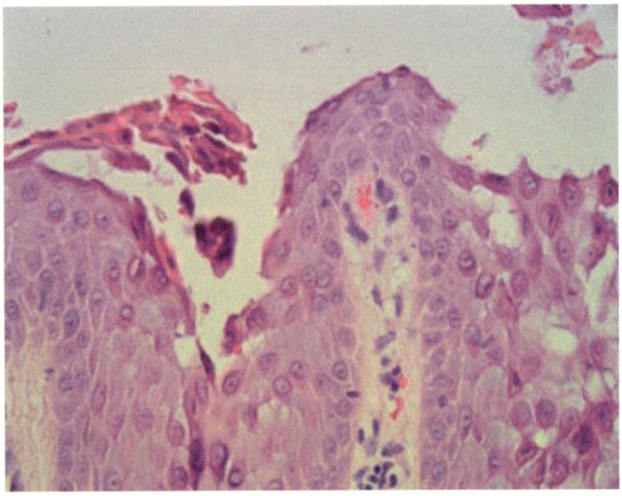

Figure 8. High power view of a skin biopsy from a patient with pemphigus foliaceus showing clefting with acantholysis and spongiosis (hematoxylin and eosin staining).

cence shows intercellular immunoglobulin G (IgG) throughout the epidermis as a result of deposition of both anti-desmoglein-1 and -3 antibodies (Figure 9). Approximately 50% of biopsies may display complement 3 (C3) [36]. In contrast, PF is characterized by both intercellular IgG and C3 predominantly in the upper half of the epidermis due to the increased density of desmoglein-1 and subsequent antibody deposition in the superficial epidermis. The diagnostic sensitivity of direct immunofluorescence in pemphigus disease is 80-95% [38].

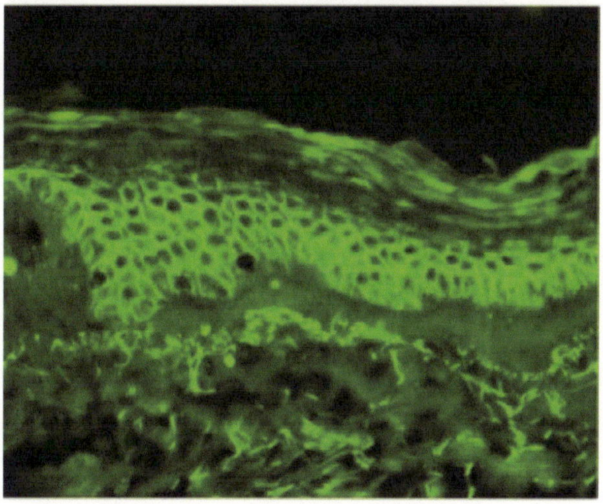

Figure 9. Direct immunofluorescence of a skin biopsy from a patient with pemphigus vulgaris revealing deposition of IgG throughout the epidermis resulting in a chicken wire appearance.

5.3. Indirect immunofluorescence

The target of pemphigus is desmoglein. Desmoglein-1 and -3 are restricted to stratified squamous epithelium, whereas desmoglein-2 is expressed in all desmosome possessing tissues [8]. In indirect immunofluorescence, patient serum is incubated with epithelial substrates containing the target antigen. In pemphigus, the most frequently used substrates are monkey esophagus, which is more sensitive for the detection of PV autoantibodies, and guinea pig esophagus and rabbit lip mucosa, which are more sensitive for the diagnosis of PF [39]. In PV, indirect immunofluorescence produces a characteristic chicken-wire pattern predominantly on the lowermost epithelial layers. The result is invariably positive in active disease. PF autoantibodies produce a chicken wire pattern in the superficial epithelial layers (Figure 10). The positivity rate is approximately 79-90% [38]. False positives can result from patient serum containing antibodies to cell surface antigens[39]; antibodies can be found in patients with staphylococcal scalded skin, penicillin adverse drug reactions, toxic epidermolysis necrosis, and burns. Importantly, patients with blood group O who have antibodies to blood groups A and B may give low false positives on indirect immunofluorescence testing, which is avoided by preabsorbing their sera with these blood group antigens. Indirect immunofluorescence titers can be used as a marker of disease activity in patients[38],[40].

6. Enzyme-Linked Immunosorbent Assay (ELISA)

Indirect immunofluorescence is not reactive with all pemphigus sera and does not differentiate between desmoglein-3 and desmoglein-1[41]. In response, ELISAs have been developed using the recombinant ectodomains of desmoglein-1 and -3 [42]. In commercially available assays,

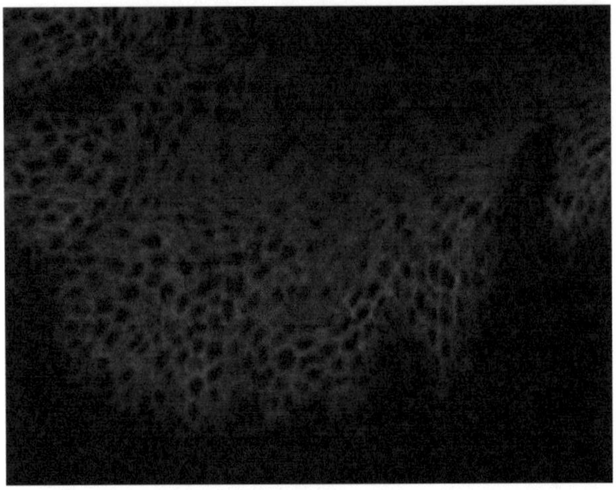

Figure 10. Indirect immunofluorescence with the serum of a patient with pemphigus foliaceus and monkey oesophagus substrate reveals deposition of specific IgG in the intercellular cement space substance of the epidermis resulting in a chicken wire appearance. There is an increased deposition in the upper layers of the epidermis.

these desmoglein ectodomains have been expressed in insect cells (MBL, Nagoya, Japan), or in human HEK293 cells (Euroimmun, Lubeck, Germany) [43]. Meta-analyses suggest that available ELISAs are highly sensitive and specific, and has a higher diagnostic accuracy than indirect immunofluorescence [44]. The quantification of these autoantibodies is useful in monitoring disease activity because the titre of circulating autoantibodies has been observed to correlate with disease activity. Specifically, the level of desmoglein-1 antibodies matches the severity of skin disease, and the level of desmoglein-3 reflects the severity of mucosal disease [45],[46].

7. Treatment

Therapy has resulted in a drastic decline of the mortality from pemphigus rate to below 7% [24],[47]; however, mortality still occurs, predominantly iatrogenic, caused by complications of the immunosuppressive therapy [24],[47]. PF tends to have a relatively benign course compared with PV. However, mortality rates of untreated endemic PF are still very high, ranging from 40 to 60% [48],[49]. With appropriate treatment endemic PF has a mortality rate of less than 10% [48]. The mortality of PV was 75% before the introduction of corticosteroids in the early 1950s [47]. Studies that differentiate PV according to clinical phenotype have shown a lower mortality in patients with predominantly mucosal PV (1–17%) compared with those with mucocutaneous PV (34–42%)[24]. Hence, the goal of managing patients with pemphigus is inducing and maintaining remission using those evidenced-based treatments that have a favourable side effect profile.

Pemphigus is a rare disease and therefore it is not surprising that only a few blinded randomized controlled trials have been performed to guide treatment decisions. A 2009 Cochrane review [50] assessed interventions for PV and PF and concluded that there is inadequate information available to ascertain optimal therapy for pemphigus. They ascertained that the quality of most studies was not high and the majority examine patients with newly diagnosed or active disease. Another consideration in the evaluation of data is lack of generally accepted definitions and measurements for the clinical evaluation of patients with pemphigus and the definitions of disease control and remission. A recent consensus statement has been released to assist with future trials enabling improved comparisons to be made [51].

As high-dose systemic corticosteroids, followed by alternate immune-suppressive agents, serves as the mainstay of initial therapy for PV, there is the need to exclude underlying latent infectious diseases that can be reactivated by the corticosteroids (e.g.: HIV, Hepatitis B and C, and tuberculosis). In addition, screening for the diseases initiated or exacerbated by high-dose 'steroids, such as hypertension, diabetes mellitus and osteoporosis is prudent.

8. Systemic corticosteroids

Systemic corticosteroids are currently the mainstay of treatment as they have a rapid onset of action and are effective in controlling disease and improving prognosis [52]. However significant side effects such as diabetes, osteoporosis, adrenal suppression, peptic ulceration, weight gain, increased susceptibility to infection, mood changes, proximal myopathy, Cushing's syndrome, and cataracts limit their usefulness. Adjuvant treatments have therefore been introduced as steroid sparing agents. Various corticosteroid regimens are used to treat pemphigus, the most common of which is a gradual reduction of an oral formulation [47]. In newly diagnosed patients, an initial daily dose of 0.5 mg/kg of prednisone/prednisolone, (or equivalent) appears preferable to 1 mg/kg. A randomized trial compared these two regimens in 19 patients with PV and 3 with PF followed for 5 years, with remission defined as less than 15 mg of corticosteroids per day to maintain disease control [53]. No difference was observed in remission or the incidence of complications between the high and low dose regimens. In a randomized trial that included only patients with newly diagnosed PV, pulsed oral dexamethasone provided no additional benefit to the combination of oral prednisone and azathioprine with remission defined as cessation of systemic treatment [54]. Furthermore, there were an increased number of adverse events in those participants receiving pulsed dexamethasone. However, the possible benefit of high dose pulsed intravenous corticosteroids in achieving disease control and maintaining remission was suggested in a small case-controlled retrospective study of patients with PV initially unresponsive to low dose of prednisone (less than 40 mg daily) [55] and an open study of new diagnosed PV patients [56]. There have no studies to date examining the effects of high dose pulsed intravenous corticosteroids in PF.

Currently no optimal regimen for corticosteroid therapy has been defined for the treatment of pemphigus despite its proven benefits. Hence in routine practice, a tailored regime is recommended. A starting dose of prednisolone 0.5 mg/kg daily is prudent that may need to be increased, until no new blister formation is observed. Such higher doses of corticosteroids including pulsed therapy may be warranted in newly diagnosed severe disease and recalcitrant disease but this remains to be substantiated in randomized studies.

9. Adjuvant treatment of pemphigus

Immunosuppressive therapy for pemphigus includes azathioprine, mycophenolate mofetil, methotrexate, cyclophosphamide, cyclosporin and dapsone. Adjuvant agents with immunomodulatory activity that have also been used in pemphigus include calcineurin inhibitors, epidermal derived growth factor and tetracycline antibiotics. The main role of these immunosuppressive medications is to function as a steroid-sparing agent. As they generally have a slow mode of onset, approximately 4-6 weeks, they are used in maintenance therapy rather than in the initiation of disease control. However, their role needs to be further elucidated as there has been only limited number of randomized controlled trials with most of the literature derived from case series reports.

9.1. Azathioprine

Azathioprine is a purine antimetabolite that is cleaved to 6-mercaptopurine, which in turn is converted to additional metabolites that inhibit *de novo* purine synthesis. Cell proliferation is inhibited and as a consequence a variety of lymphocyte functions are impaired. Azathioprine is commonly used to treat pemphigus; a survey of dermatologists in 2003 showed it was the most commonly prescribed adjuvant agent used to treat PV [57]. It has even been used as monotherapy in mild cases [58]. In a recent randomized trial conducted by Chams-Davatchi et al, 120 new patients with PV were treated for over one year with one of four regimens. These regimes were prednisolone alone, prednisolone plus azathioprine, prednisolone plus intravenous cyclophosphamide and prednisolone plus mycophenolate mofetil [59]. Azathioprine reduced the cumulative dose of prednisolone compared with prednisolone alone however remission rates were similar. Side effects were similar between the two groups. Thus in this trial, which included only patients with PV, azathioprine reduced the cumulative corticosteroid dose but not the rate of remission. More recently, a non-randomized study compared high dose oral prednisone daily (1.5 mg/kg/daily) versus low dose oral prednisone (40 mg on alternate days) plus azathioprine (100 mg/daily) in 36 patients with oral PV [60]. Both treatments resulted in high rates of clinical remission; the monotherapy group showed a reduced mean time to remission but this group was associated with an increased rate of treatment-associated adverse events Other non-randomized trials using azathioprine are have generally shown favourable outcomes in PV [61],[62].

9.2. Mycophenolate mofetil

Mycophenolate mofetil is a prodrug and its active drug, mycophenolic acid, inhibits inosine monophosphate dehydrogenase, an important enzyme in guanine nucleotide synthesis. Lymphocytes are highly dependent on this pathway and are selectively inhibited by mycophenolate mofetil [63]. In the randomized trial by Chams-Davatchi et al, no difference in remission was observed for mycophenolate mofetil when compared to prednisolone alone [59]. In this same study no difference in remission was demonstrated between azathioprine and mycophenolate mofetil. The steroid sparing effect of mycophenolate mofetil was inferior to azathioprine. Beissert et al. compared oral methylprednisolone plus azathioprine with mycophenolate mofetil in 33 patients with PV and 7 patients with PF [64]. The primary outcome was complete healing of all lesions. This study concluded that mycophenolate mofetil and azathioprine demonstrated similar efficacy. Safety profiles were similar as was corticosteroid-sparing effects. There were less severe side effects observed in the mycophenolate group but this was not statistically significant. Many non-randomized trials have supported the use of mycophenolate mofetil in the treatment of pemphigus [65]-[69]. The majority of patients in these trials had PV. Mycophenolate mofetil is generally well tolerated; lymphopenia, gastro-intestinal symptoms and infections are the most common side effects. Currently it is a relatively expensive medication, often precluding its off-label use. The drug is usually commenced at dose of 1 g per day in adult patients, and if required, increased in 500-mg increments up to doses of 2-3 g per day [70].

9.3. Cyclophosphamide

Cyclophosphamide is an alkylating agent that disturbs DNA synthesis and cell division. Cyclophosphamide interferes with DNA integrity and function inducing cell death in rapidly proliferating tissues including lymphocytes. This provides the basis for their therapeutic and toxic properties. Several randomized trials have assessed cyclophosphamide in treatment of pemphigus. Chrysomallis et al. used oral cyclophosphamide in patients with PV whose disease was limited to oral involvement [71]. Twenty-eight patients were divided into 3 groups and given corticosteroids alone, corticosteroids with cyclophosphamide or cyclosporine. No difference in remission was seen when cyclophosphamide was compared with corticosteroids alone, and at 5 years, all patients had their disease controlled with a low dose corticosteroid regimen. The more recent study by Chams-Davatchi et al. described above and comprising entirely of patients with PV concluded that there was no difference in remission rates following pulsed intravenous cyclophosphamide therapy [59]. A randomized control trial that included 6 patients with PF as well as 16 with PV compared pulsed cyclophosphamide with dexamethasone and daily cyclophosphamide with methylprednisolone plus azathioprine [72]. No difference in disease control was observed for the cyclophosphamide group compared to the azathioprine group after 2 years. Several non-randomized case series have utilized pulse cyclophosphamide with variable outcomes [73]-[75].

Given the lack of superiority of cyclophosphamide over other regimes in randomized trials and its well-described serious side effect profile, the authors recommend that its use be restricted for the treatment of severe or refractory cases of PF, where alternative agents such as rituximab or IVIg are not available.

9.4. Cyclosporin

Cyclosporin is a calcineurin inhibitor that prevents dephosphorylation of nuclear factor of activated T cells (NFAT) preventing its translocation into nucleus and as a consequence the T cells fail to respond to specific antigenic stimulation. Cyclosporin also increases expression of TGF- beta, a potent inhibitor of IL-2–stimulated T-cell proliferation. A randomized trial compared oral methylprednisolone alone with oral methylprednisolone plus cyclosporin in 33 newly diagnosed patients, 29 with PV and 4 with PF [76]. The patients were followed for

4-6 years and the investigators concluded that the combination regimen of corticosteroids and cyclosporin provided no additional benefit over corticosteroids alone. Side effects, including hypertrichosis, hypertension and renal dysfunction, were more common in the cyclosporin group. The randomized controlled study by Chrysomallis et al. in newly diagnosed PV limited to oral involvement found no difference in remission or relapse rates between the cyclophosphamide and cyclosporine (5 mg/kg) groups [71]. Again, adverse events were more common in the cyclosporin group and included hypertrichosis and renal impairment. A case series reported successful the successful treatment of 6 patients with recalcitrant PV [77].

The randomized trials have not supported the use of cyclosporine at a dose of 5 mg/kg for the treatment of new onset pemphigus and side effects are relatively common. Further randomized controlled trials are required to determine its benefit in recalcitrant disease.

9.5. Dapsone

Dapsone has anti-inflammatory and antimicrobial actions. Its immunomodulatory action is incompletely understood but several actions have been described including prevention of the respiratory burst from myeloperoxidase, suppression of neutrophil migration by blocking integrin-mediated adherence, inhibition of adherence of antibodies to neutrophils, and reduction of eicosanoid release. Most studies utilising dapsone have been performed in patients with PV. A randomized controlled trial performed in 19 patients, all with PV, compared dapsone with placebo [78]. Patients were in the maintenance phase after glucocorticoids and/or cytotoxic agents (azathioprine, mycophenolate or methotrexate) were used to achieve remission. Doses of dapsone were increased to 150 mg per day and then to a further 200 mg per day if tolerated. The trial was performed over 1 year, and the main outcome measured was reduction of prednisolone to doses of 7.5mg/day or less. Five of the 9 patients in the placebo group achieved the main outcome compared with 3 out of 10 in the placebo group. The difference was not statistically significant although there was a trend favouring dapsone as a steroid sparing agent. A retrospective study in 9 patients with PV suggested that dapsone reduced steroid dependence in these patients [79]. Another study reported improvement in 5 of 9 cases of superficial pemphigus treated with dapsone [80]. A recent meta-analysis comprising 55 patients with pemphigus revealed that 32 patients with PV and 14 patients with PF responded to dapsone [81].

The side effects of dapsone observed in these studies include methaemoglobinaemia, haemolysis and agranulocytosis. [81],[82] Patients should be tested for glucose-6-phosphate dehydrogenase deficiency prior to commencing this agent. Dapsone at best may have a role as a steroid sparing agent in the maintaining remission in pemphigus but cannot be recommended in treatment of acute disease.

9.6. Methotrexate

The antimetabolite methotrexate is a folic acid analogue that competitively inhibits dihydrofolate reductase and has multiple immunosuppressive actions including suppressing lymphocytes in the skin [83],[84]. A small number of non-randomized trials have investigated the

http://dx.doi.org/10.5772/56423

role of methotrexate in treatment of pemphigus. The most recent study [83] treated 9 patients with chronic active PV, who were unable to successfully wean their prednisolone dose. They were treated with a mean dose of 12.5 mg per week of methotrexate. Prednisolone was discontinued in 6 of the 9 patients within 6 months of commencing methotrexate. There were minimal adverse effects reported in the study. A recent review of the English literature revealed that 111 (82%) of 136 pemphigus patients responded to methotrexate [85]. However, meaningful conclusions are limited by the lack of randomized trials, varying doses and schedules of treatment, and insufficient information on clinical progress including the lack of consistency of the length of follow up.

Thus methotrexate may be useful as a steroid sparing agent but further trials are required before recommending methotrexate as an initial steroid-sparing agent.

Medication	Dose	Contra-indications	Pre-Therapeutic Investigations	Monitoring	Adverse Reactions
Corticosteroids ("steroids")	prednisolone: (1) ½-1 mg per kg/ bodyweight of the patient for 4 days (or longer in pemphigus) with rapid taper until clinical remission occurs (2) < 7.5 mg/daily	• Active infectious diseases: Tb, HIV, HBV, HCV	• Tb, HIV, HBV, HCV	Systemic: • hypertension, psychosis, diabetes mellitus, weight gain, cataracts Oral Mucosa: • candidiasis, mucosal atrophy	hypertension, psychosis, diabetes mellitus, weight gain, cataracts Oral Mucosa: candidiasis, mucosal atrophy
Calcineurin-Inhibitors: pimecrolimus (Elidel®)	<u>Topical Application Only:</u> thin layer to affected mucosa twice daily	A *causal* relationship has <u>not</u> been established with malignancy. Skin cancer and lymphoma have been reported in patients treated with topical calcineurin inhibitors, including pimecrolimus 1% cream.			irritation, pruritis and erythema on application
Lysosomotropic Amines: hydroxyl-chloroquine (Plaquenil®)	200-400 mg (once daily)	• pre-existing retinopathy • psoriasis • porphyria • G6PD deficiency	• baseline visual acuity testing (for macular degeneration) by an Ophthalmologist • FBC; G6DP levels; LFT's	• annual baseline visual acuity testing • FBC and LFT's weekly for first 4 weeks; thereafter, only if indicated	UV (sun) light–initiated lichenoid cutaneous reactions Note: slow onset of action of up to 3 months
azathioprine (Imuran®)	1.0-2.0 mg per kg bodyweight/daily (once daily)	• recent use of live vaccines • pregnancy (Category D) (including partner of male patient) • concomitant allopurinol	• thiopurine methyl-transferase (TPMT) assay (determines risk of bone marrow aplasia) • FBC; LFT's; E/U/C	• FBC weekly for first 8 weeks; thereafter monthly	severe adverse reaction with xanthine oxidase inhibitors of which the most potent is allopurinol (Progout® Zyloprim®)

mycophenolate (CellCept®, Myfortic®)	max 2 g/day (once daily or divided dose)	• pregnancy (Category D)	• HIV, HBV, HCV	• FBC and LFT's weekly for first 4 weeks; thereafter, only if indicated	malignancy risk eg skin cancer, lymphoma; infection; progressive multifocal leuco-encephalopathy; bone marrow depression
dapsone (Dapsone®)	maintenance dose: 50-100 mg daily (≥ 300 mg daily		• FBC, G6DP levels, LFT's • HIV, HBV, HCV	• FBC, LFT's weekly for the first month, monthly for six months and semi-annually thereafter	dose related haemolysis, especially in G6DP deficient patients; agranulocytosis; toxic hepatitis and cholestatic jaundice
methotrexate (Methoblastin®)	10 to 25 mg/ ***WEEKLY ONLY*** until adequate response is achieved	• pregnancy (Category D) • liver/renal impairment • HIV, HBV, HCV • immune-deficiency; • concomitant retinoinds	FBC, LFT's, E/U/C HIV, HBV, HCV	• FBC weekly for first 8 weeks, thereafter monthly	hepato/ nephrotoxicity; ulcerative stomatitis; bone marrow depression; immune-suppression
Rituximab (Mabthera®)	375 mg/m² (body surface area) once weekly for 4 weeks or 2x 1.0g -500 mg ivi infusions over two weeks	• Murine(mouse) protein hypersensitivity	• Tb, HIV, HBV, HCV	• infection	progressive multifocal leucoencephalopathy (PML)

(A)

Medication	Actions
corticosteroids (" 'steroids)	Profound, generalised inhibitory effects on inflammatory processes and cells achieved by the control of protein synthesis by reacting with certain corticosteroid responsive genes of sensitive cells in many tissues: ⇩ production of acute inflammatory mediators, especially eicosonoids, postaglndins and leukotrienes. (corticosteroids increase the production of a polypeptide – *lipocortin,* that in turn inhibits phospholipase A_2 the enzyme responsible for the mobilising arachniodonic acid from cell membranes) ⇩ production and numbers of circulating immune-competent cells: e.g.: neutrophils, macrophages, T and B lymphocytes ⇩ Complement activation ⇩ activity of macrophages and fibroblasts involved in the chronic stages of inflammation – leading to decreased inflammation and healing
cyclosporine tacrolimus	Calcineurin inhibitors:

http://dx.doi.org/10.5772/56423

pimecrolimus	•binds to the cytosolic protein cyclophilin of T-lymphocytes and the complex of cyclosporin (or other calcineurin-inhibitor) and cyclophilin inhibits calcineurin, which normally induces the transcription of interleukin-2. ⇩ lymphokine production and interleukin release (further reducing the function of effector T-cells)
hydroxyl-chloroquine (Plaquenil®)	Lipophilic weak base that passes easily through plasma membranes to accumulate in acidic vesicles, such as the lysosomes of the inflammatory cells and acts by: ⇩ antigen presentation by the antigen-presenting cells (APC's) ⇩ cytokine production (e.g.: Tumour Necrosis Factor-alpha (TNF-α), Interleukin-6 (IL-6), Interferon-gamma (IFN-γ)) ⇩ stimulation of the toll-like receptors • prostaglandin antagonist
azathioprine (Imuran®)	Azathioprine is an imidazole derivative of 6-mercaptopurine (6-MP) into which is rapidly broken down (in vivo). • 6-MP readily crosses cell membranes and is converted intracellularly into a number of purine thioanalogues, including the main active nucleotide: thioinosinic acid. • thioinosinic acid inhibits many pathways in nucleic acid biosynthesis causing damage to deoxyribonucleic acid (DNA), through incorporation of this "false" purine thio-analogue. • this action is restricted to the cells involved in determination and amplification of immune response; the B and T lymphocytes as they are unable to source alternate or extrinsic nucleotides being entirely dependent for their proliferation on de novo synthesis of purines, whereas other cell types can utilise salvage pathways.
mycophenolate (CellCept®, Myfortic®)	Mycophenolic acid (MPA) is a potent, selective, uncompetitive and reversible inhibitor of inosine monophosphate dehydrogenase (IMPDH) which inhibits the de novo pathway of guanosine nucleotide synthesis but without incorporation into the cell's DNA: • MPA has more potent cytostatic effects on T and B lymphocytes than on other cells because these cells are entirely dependent for their proliferation on their *de novo* synthesis of purines, whereas other cell types can utilise salvage pathways • depletion of guanosine nucleotides also leads to the inhibition of glycosylation of the adhesion molecules on lymphocytes further interfering in their immune functions
dapsone (Dapsone®)	Dapsone is effective in dermatoses with abnormal neutrophil accumulation • Dapsone interferes in chemotactic-mediated migration of neutrophils and neutrophil function by: (1) inactivating the function of the G-protein (Gi type) that initiates the signal transduction cascade common to chemotactic stimuli; (2) the cytokine mediated adherence of neutrophils to the vascular endothelial cells; and (3) inhibits neutrophil MPO-mediated iodination and cytotoxicity and eosinophil peroxidise, thereby, dapsone suppresses neutrophil recruitment and protects cells from neutrophil- and eosinophil-mediated injury by directly inhibiting the generation of toxic, oxygen-derived radicals. • in antibody mediated diseases, dapsone appears to interfere in the adherence of neutrophils to the auto-antigenic antibodies (IgA and IgG) bound to the various target sites in the basement membrane zone, so protecting the epithelial cells from neutrophil-derived cytolytic agents ⇩ release of prostaglandins and leukotrienes and so blocks their inflammatory effects
methotrexate (Methoblastin®)	Antimetabolite cytotoxin. Methotrexate (MTX) competitively inhibits the enzyme *dihydrofolate reductase* and so prevents the regeneration of intermediates (such as tetrahydrofolate) essential for the synthesis of purines and thymidylate so preventing DNA synthesis: • actively proliferating tissues such as the bone marrow stem cells, dermal epithelium, and lymphocytes (as well as the oral mucosal cells) are in general more sensitive to the effects of MTX • MTX has more potent cytostatic effects on T and B lymphocytes than on other cells because these cells are entirely dependent for their proliferation on their *de novo* synthesis of purines, whereas other cell types can utilise salvage pathways

Rituximab (Mabthera®)	Rituximab is a genetically engineered chimeric murine/human monoclonal antibody that binds specifically to the antigen CD20, a transmembrane molecule located on pre-B and mature B-lymphocytes, only. This non-glycosylated phosphoprotein is found on both normal (and malignant B cells), *but* not on haemopoietic stem cells, pro-B cells, normal plasma cells or other normal tissues:
	• inhibits CD20 which regulates the early steps in the activation process for B-cell cycle initiation and differentiation • the depletion of circulating autoreactive B cells (for up to 12 months) and , presumably specific downregulation of dsg3-specific CD4(+ve) T-lymphocytes and the associated release of proinflammatory cytokines mayre-establish immune homeostasis and tolerance
	(B)

A: Tb = tuberculosis, HIV = human immune-deficiency virus, HBV = hepatitis B virus, HCV = hepatitis C virus, G6DP = glucose-6-phosphate dehydrogenase, FBC – full blood count, LFT's = liver function tests, UV = ultraviolet light, E/U/C = electrolytes/urea/creatinine

B: ⇩ = decreased or reduced

Table 2. (A) Therapeutic Agents Useful in the treatment of Pemphigus, (B) Therapeutic Agents Useful in Treating of Pemphigus

9.7. Gold

Auad [86] performed a blinded placebo-controlled randomized trial on the utility of auranofin in 30 patients with PF. Nearly one third of the patients withdrew from the active treatment arm due to side effects. In the placebo group, a reduction in the mean corticosteroid steroid dose was evident. Other case series comprising patients with PV and/or PF have described similar findings [87]-[89]. The most recent study published showed that 62% of patients with PV achieved remission or halve their dose of prednisone during a period of 10 years of intramuscular gold therapy [90]. However, the mean time to halve the dose of prednisone was 3 months and 42% developed side effects blood dyscrasia, proteinuria and nephrotic syndrome, cutaneous reactions and dizziness. These adverse effects in addition to the relatively long time to take effect as a steroid-sparing agent preclude its use in favour of other steroid-sparing agents in the treatment of treatment of pemphigus.

9.8. Tetracycline antibiotics and nicotinamide

Tetracycline antibiotics with and without nicotinamide have been combined with other adjuvant agents as treatment for pemphigus. Several small non-randomized trials have shown varying results [91]-[93]. Minocycline given at a dose of 100 mg per day allowed the reduction of prednisolone in 6 out of 10 patients with pemphigus [91]. Tetracycline at a dose of 2 g per day for 1 month reducing to 1 g per day for 4 weeks enabled more rapid tapering of corticosteroids in 13 patients with PV [93]. However the study by Alspoy found that a combination of tetracycline (2 g/d) and nicotinamide (1.5 g/d) for 2 months was not an effective alternative to the classic forms of therapy in 14 patients with pemphigus [92]. Further trials are needed before recommending these agents.

9.9. Topical agents

9.9.1. Epidermal growth factor

A double-blind randomized controlled study investigated the use of epidermal growth factor (EGF) on skin lesions of 20 patients with PV [94]. Topical epidermal growth factor 10 ug/g in 0.1% silver sulfadiazine cream was applied to skin lesions daily until lesions had healed and compared to the effect of applying 0.1% silver sulfadiazine (SSD) cream alone. Topical EGF appeared to hasten lesion healing by a median of 6 days compared to SSD.

9.9.2. Topical corticosteroids (Clobetasol)

A small study comprised of 4 patients with mild PF and 3 with mild PV were treated with the very potent topical corticosteroid, Clobetasol propionate 0.05%, as a sole agent [95]. The cream was applied to mucosal lesions and involved skin twice a day for at least 15 days, then progressively tapered. Control of disease was defined as healing of lesions was obtained, with a 75% decrease in the number of new lesions per week without the addition of systemic treatment. Disease control was achieved in all 7 patients, with cutaneous remission attained in 15 days, although mucosal regression occurring more slowly. In 4 patients, remission was maintained with topical corticosteroid alone for a mean 19-month follow up. In 3 patients, relapse occurred after 2-11 months, requiring systemic treatment. Another study is in progress comparing the effect of Clobetosol with placebo in pemphigus vulgaris.

9.9.3. Topical calcineurin inhibitors

Tacrolimus and Pimecrolimus are non-steroidal immunomodulatory macrobactams that inhibit the enzyme, calcineurin, impairing the production and IL-2 and subsequent T-cell activation and proliferation [96]. A small number of case reports and case series suggest a useful role for Tacrolimus in mild PV and PF but further randomized controlled trials are required to clarify its role in this setting [97]-[99]. A recent double blind study of 11 patients with PV refractory to azathioprine and corticosteroids showed a marked response to pimecrolimus 1% by day 15 when compared to placebo using the epithelialization index [100].

10. Novel therapies and strategies

10.1. Biological agents

10.1.1. Rituximab

Rituximab is a chimeric (human/murine) monoclonal antibody directed against CD20, a cell surface molecule specific to B cells. Although it was initially approved for use in B-cell non-Hodgkin's lymphoma, a growing number of reports have described the efficacy of rituximab for B-cell depletion in the treatment of autoimmune diseases [101]. The mode of action of rituximab in autoimmune diseases includes the removal of precursors of autoantibody-producing plasma cells, and impairment of autoantigen presentation to CD4 cells [102]. In PV, Eming et al, show that rituximab not also causes marked reduction of anti-desmoglein 3 antibodies but also depletion of desmoglein-specific CD4 cells. In contrast, tetanus toxoid-specific CD4 cells were not affected nor were the overall number of CD4 cells [103]. Tetaus toxoid has been used in as an antigen in the assessment of memory CD4 cell responses [104]. Eming et al, speculate that this specific effect of rituximab on autoreactive rather than pathogen-specific T cells is that the latter do not require CD20 B cells as antigen-presenting cells. A number of case reports and series have demonstrated the benefit on the use of rituximab in over 40 patients with either PV or PF [40]'[105]-[115]. The largest case series to date comprising 42 patients, 37 with PV and 5 with PF, utilized the rheumatoid arthritis protocol where two 1g infusions of rituximab are administered 15 days apart [116]. Patients were followed for up to 5 years and 36 of the 42 patients achieved a complete response and were able to cease corticosteroids within 6 months from induction therapy. Twenty patients experienced relapses with the time to relapse ranging from 8 to 64 months. Relapses were treated with rituximab (500 mg) without corticosteroids resulting in a new complete response. Importantly, no serious adverse events were observed.

The largest case series to date using the lymphoma protocol where rituximab is administered weekly (375 mg/m^2) for 4 weeks induced remission in 12 of 14 patients with PV and 6 of 7 patients with PF within 3 months [117]. These patients had previously not responded to first-line immunosuppressive agents or had contraindications to corticosteroid therapy. The treatment was generally well tolerated; however, two cases were complicated by severe infection, one resulting in death. Similarly, Canchini et al, showed that the administration of rituximab, 375 mg/m^2 once weekly for 4 weeks, induced remission in all 10 patients with PV and both patients with PF [118]. Another study comprising 11 patients with refractory PV, evaluated the effect of combination therapy consisting of 10 infusions of rituximab (375 mg/m^2) and 6 infusions of intravenous immunoglobulin (IVIg) (2 g/kg body weight) administered over a 6-month period [119]. Remission was induced in 9 patients for a period of 22 to 37 months following treatment and there were no reports of serious adverse events.

More recently, Kasperkiewicz et al reported use of rituximab in combination with immunoadsorption, pulsed dexamethasone and azathioprine or mycophenolate mofetil in 23 patients. [120] IA was performed at initially 3- and later 4-week intervals until lesions healed by 90%; 1 g rituximab was given at weeks 1 and 3, and intravenous dexamethasone pulses were administered at first every 3 weeks and then at increasing intervals in addition to daily azathioprine or mycophenolate mofetil. All patients demonstrated clinical improvement within the first few weeks of therapy accompanies by a concomitant rapid fall in anti-desmoglein antibody levels. However, two patients had non -atal severe adverse events; one developed *Staphylococcus aureus* sepsis from a central intravenous line followed by spinal haemorrhage and transient paraplegia, and another developed extensive herpes simplex infection

The high frequency of treatment failure with corticosteroids and first line immunosuppressive therapies has raised the issue of whether rituximab should be implemented earlier in the treatment of PV. Horvath et al conducted a study comprising 15 patients (12 with PV, 3 with

PF) who were treated with two infusions of rituximab (500 mg each) at an interval of 2 weeks [121]. All 15 patients responded to therapy. Eight patients achieved complete remission in a median period of 5 weeks. Seven patients achieved partial remission in a median period of 34 5 weeks. Relapses (40%) were seen between 53 and 103 weeks after start of therapy.

In the majority of these studies, abrogation of peripheral B cells and concomitant reduction in the level of circulating antipemphigus autoantibodies for 6 to 12 months occurs with only two to four infusions of rituximab. Interestingly, clinical remission in both PV and PF is often sustained beyond B cell recovery. The reason as provided Mouquet et al, is that the phenotype of restored B cells following rituximab treatment is that of a naïve B cell with a diverse repertoire rather than a primed autoreactive B cell [122].

Accumulation of the data from case reports and series reveals that 16% of patients with PV developed the serious complications of bacterial sepsis, fatal *Pneumocystis jirovecii* pneumonia, persistent hypogammaglobulinemia or pulmonary embolism [123]. Concerns have also been raised regarding the role of rituximab and other biological agents used in patients with other immune-mediated diseases such as rheumatoid arthritis developing Progressive Multifocal Leukoencephalopathy (PML) [124]. PML is an inevitably fatal demyelinating disease of the central nervous system, that occurs almost exclusively in immunosuppressed individuals due to reactivation of the polyomavirus JC (JCV) [125]. This is in contrast to rarity of adverse events observe in patients treated for non-Hodgkin's lymphoma [126]. Although, the question has been raised of the use of rituximab as a first line agent due to the impressive rates of remission [127], the incidence of serious side effects may at present preclude its role in initial therapy. Ongoing surveillance of patients treated with rituximab for pemphigus and other autoimmune diseases is required to monitor for long-term complications.

There is enough evidence to suggest that rituximab should be the therapy of choice for patients with pemphigus who have refractory disease or contraindications to first-line immunosuppressive therapy although randomized controlled trials have not been performed and as such, there is no uniform protocol on its administration. The value of adjunctive therapies such as IVIg and IA in patients treated with rituximab for pemphigus needs to be also further elucidated. However, one of the most important questions to address is whether it is cost effective and safe to administer rituximab for PV and severe PF as a first line agent.

10.1.2. TNF-antagonists

Studies have demonstrated that TNF released by keratinocytes plays a role in acantholysis in PV. Human keratinocytes pretreated with anti-TNF antibodies, are resistant to the acantholytic effect of anti-desmoglein 3 antibodies [128],[129]. Furthermore, TNF-deficient mice are more susceptible to blister formation after injection with anti-desmoglein 3 antibodies [128]. The role of TNF in PF has not been as extensively studied. Etanercept [130]-[133], infliximab [134],[135], and adalimumab [136], have all demonstrated benefit in a small number of patients with refractory PV. Randomized controlled trials of infliximab and etanercept in refractory PV are currently in progress. However, the effect of these agents in refractory PF has not been reported to date.

10.2. Intravenous immunoglobulin

IVIg is a fractionated and purified blood product derived from the pooled plasma of up to 15, 000 healthy donors. Hence it has a high concentration of IgG with a broad range of specificities against various antigens [137]. The mode of action of IVIg in autoimmune disease has not been clearly defined but is probably multifactorial and includes provision of anti-idiotypic antibodies, modulation of expression and function of Fc receptors thereby neutralizing the effect of pathogenic antibodies, blocking of complement activation, reduced secretion of pro-inflammatory cytokines through modulation of dendritic, T and B-cell activation [138],[139]. IVIg upregulates endogenous caspase inhibitors protecting keratinocytes from proapoptotic molecules and thereby inhibits acantholysis [140]. In PV, IVIg causes a selective and rapid decline in serum levels of pathogenic antibodies, specifically IgG1 and IgG4 anti-desmoglein-1 and anti-desmoglein-3 antibodies without affecting total serum IgG levels [141],[142]. A reduction in anti-desmoglein-1 antibodies also occurs in PF [143]. FcRn receptors, which normally function to protect serum IgG from degredation, are saturated following IVIg resulting in catabolism of all IgG molecules including autoreactive antibodies [144]. However, pathogenic autoantibodies are selectively reduced because catabolized normal antibodies are replaced by those present in the IVIg preparation [141].

Three case series and 1 retrospective analysis comprising 54 patients with refractory PV documented the induction of clinical remission following IVIg in all but 2 patients [145]-[148]. Two case series involving a total of 15 patients with refractory PF all responded to IVIg [149], [150]. One of these studies featuring 7 patients revealed a prolonged mean remission time of 18.6 months following discontinuation of IVIg [150]. Two retrospective analyses that included 17 patients with refractory PV and 2 patients with refractory PF, however, demonstrated a much less favourable response with the majority of patients harbouring active disease following IVIg [151],[152]. Recently, a double blind randomized study investigated the effect of a 5 day course of IVIg at varying doses (400, 200 or 0 mg/kg/day) in 40 patients with PV and 21 patients with PF resistant to doses of steroids greater that 20 mg daily [153]. The study did not specify whether these patients had previously been treated with or were currently receiving corticosteroid-sparing immunosuppressive agents. The patients were maintained on their study entry dose of corticosteroids for the duration of the trial. The primary end point was the time to escape from the protocol, which was defined as the length of period that the patient remained on the protocol, without any additional treatment. Patients that showed no improvement after 2 weeks or developed fresh lesions necessitating an increase in corticosteroids or additional immunosuppression were considered as having escaped from the protocol. The study demonstrated a significantly longer time to escape the protocol, and a lower disease activity index accompanied by a fall in anti-desmoglein antibody levels in the 400 mg/kg/day group at days 43 and 85 for both PV and PF patients. There were no significant differences in the side effects observed between the groups. Adverse events that were reported in a minority of patients included fever, headache, palpitations, hypertension, gastrointestinal bleeding, increased creatinine, abnormal liver function tests, and anemia. One patient in the 200 mg/kg/day died as a result of liver failure from exacerbation of pre-existing chronic hepatitis C. Hence, this study does provide useful evidence for the efficacy of IVIg in both PV and PF. Cessation

http://dx.doi.org/10.5772/56423

of IVIg may result in new synthesis of autoantibodies exceeding that initially present [154] and this rebound in antibody levels may minimized by concurrent cytotoxic therapy.

Comparative trials in refractory disease with other modalities such as biological agents and extracorporeal treatments still need to be performed. The considerable expense of IVIg warrants clarification of the optimal dose, frequency and duration of therapy. Further studies are required to determine whether IVIg can be ceased once remission is achieved, and the patient maintained on conventional first line immunosuppressive agents to minimize rebound synthesis of pathogenic antibodies.

10.3. Extracorporeal treatments

10.3.1. Plasmapheresis

Plasmapheresis results in the potential removal of pathogenic antibodies from the patient's plasma. Forty patients with pemphigus were recruited in a multicentre study and randomized to receive prednisone alone or prednisone and plasma exchange, which consisted of 10 treatments over 4 weeks [155]. No adjuvant immunosupressive therapy was used for any of the patients. No difference was observed between the 2 groups. Four patients in each group did not achieve disease control. Four patients in the plasmapheresis group died from either sepsis or thromboembolism. The lack of response is surprising as Nagasaka et al, demonstrated in 15 patients with PV and 1 patient with PF that one centrifugal plasmapheresis treatment eliminates 15% of the IgG autoantibodies as measured in the effluents and this is reflected in serum measurements performed one day later [156]. Numerous case series have demonstrated benefit in severe or recalcitrant pemphigus when plasmapheresis is combined not only with corticosteroids but other immunosuppressive agents as well [157]-[161]. Many of these patients experienced side effects including thrombocytopenia, hypocalcemia, urticaria, fever, hypotension, acute hepatitis, nausea, dizziness and leg cramps. The beneficial response observed in these case series studies in contrast to the randomized controlled study of Guillaume et al, may therefore be explained by the concurrent use of immunosuppressive agents in order to prevent the rebound production of autoantibodies. Hence further randomized control studies are needed to clarify the value of plasmapheresis combined with immunosuppressive therapy.

10.3.2. Immunoadsorption

Immunoadsorption (IA) is an extracorporeal treatment for the selective removal of antibodies and circulating immune complexes from plasma. This differs from plasmapheresis, which nonspecifically removes plasma proteins including clotting factors, hormones and albumin, thus requiring substitution of fresh frozen plasma or albumin. The Food and Drug Administration approved IA for the treatment of rheumatoid arthritis, idiopathic thrombocytopenic purpure and hemophilia with inhibitors. It has also been used off label for the treatment of various autoimmune mediated conditions including dilated cardiomyopathy, systemic lupus erythematosus, myasthenia gravis and autoimmune bullous disorders [162].

Initially, 4 case series and 2 case reports totalling 31 patients with PV and 5 patients with PF reported efficacy for IA in combination with immunosuppressive therapies in the treatment of recalcitrant disease [163]-[167]. The treatment schedule generally consisted of 3 initial cycles on consecutive days, a fourth cycle on day 8, followed by 19 cycles in incrementally prolonged intervals of 1 to 4 weeks. However, relapses are common once IA is discontinued and concurrent immunosuppressive therapy tapered [167]. More recently, a small case series comprising 7 patients with refractory PV demonstrated that 23 cycles of IA administered 40 weeks, as described above, in combination with rituximab (375 mg/m^2 weekly for 4 weeks) and concomitant conventional therapy resulted in complete remission in 3 patients for a period of between 13 and 30 months with minimal or no maintenance immunosupresion [168]. One patient attained partial remission but required significantly less dose of corticosteroids than prior to IA and rituximab. The remaining 3 patients relapsed following the completion of treatment. Two of these patients achieved remission when IVIg (2 g/kg body weight every 4 weeks) was administered and the other only partially responded to IVIg. A retrospective study on refractory PV compared the efficacy of IA in 6 patients with rituximab in 5 patients and showed remission in all patients at 6 months [169]. This remission was sustained in all patients who had received rituximab compared to half of those that received IA. Randomized trials are required to compare the efficacy of rituximab or IVIg with IA and determine any additional benefit from a combination of these modalities.

The treatment is generally well tolerated. Rare adverse events that have been reported include catheter related sepsis, *Pneumocystis jerovecii* pneumonia, mild hypotension, bradycardia and in relation to anticoagulant use, hypocalcemia and paraesthesia. The trials by Schmidt et al, and Shiminovich et al, showed that the combination of IA and immunosuppression resulted in anemia in 30% of patients [164],[167].

10.3.3. Extracorporeal Photochemotherapy (ECP)

In ECP, a patient's leukocytes are collected, exposed to 8-methoxypsoralen, irradiated with ultraviolet-A light and reinfused into the patient. The principle of ECP is to induce apoptosis of leukocytes with ultraviolet-A radiation after their presentation by psoralens [170]. Early apoptotic cells produce anti-inflammatory cytokines such as IL-10 and TGF-beta, which stimulates their engulfment by macrophages and immature dendritic cells. The further production of IL-10 and TGF-beta by these antigen presenting cells with subsequent down regulation of proinflammatory cytokines such as TNF, IL-1 and IL-12 results in immunosupression and absence of co-stimulation of effector T cells [171]. A deficiency of apoptotic cell clearance may contribute to the pathogenesis of autoimmune diseases including pemphigus and therefore ECP may enhance clearance of autoreactive cells and the reduce formation of pathogenic autoantibodies by B cells [172],[173]. Collectively, 9 patients, 8 with PV and 1 with PF, originating from a small number of case studies and series, received ECP for refractory disease in conjunction with their baseline immunosuprressive agents. [174]-[177]. In contrast to the patients with PV, the lone patient with PF achieved only partial remission and long term immunosuppression was unable to be weaned successfully [177]. ECP was well tolerated in these patients with no adverse effects reported.

10.4. Cholinergic agonists

Studies have suggested that acetylcholine and its receptors are involved in the acantholysis of pemphigus. Approximately 85% of patients with pemphigus have antibodies against acetylcholine receptors on keratinocytes [178]. Cholinergic antagonists mediate similar acantholytic effects on keratinocytes as PV IgG [179]. Acantholytic antibodies can recognize the alpha-9 acetylcholine receptor [180] and pemphaxin [181], which can function as an acetylcholine receptor. Finally, cholinergic agonists can prevent acantholysis *in vivo* [182] and reverse the process in vitro [179].

Grando demonstrated a response in 3 of 6 patients with PV treated with pyridostigmine bromide and conventional immunosuppression with 2 responders ultimately able to control their disease with pyridostigmine bromide alone [183]. A recent double blind placebo controlled study comprising 3 PV patients showed a superior epithelialisation effect from 4% pilocarpine gel compared with placebo [184]. The use of these agents in PF has not been reported.

10.5. Peptide immunotherapy

Immunization with intravenous desmoglein-3 peptides was developed to suppress production of anti-desmoglein-3 antibodies through inactivation of disease specific CD4 cells. A phase I clinical trial in PV patients found no significant change in anti-desmoglein-3 antibodies following administration of intravenous desmoglein-3 peptides [185]. Additional studies utilizing higher doses and longer treatment are in progress. It remains to be determined whether peptide immunotherapy with desmoglein-1 peptides will have a beneficial effect in PF.

10.5.1. Inhibitors of intracellular signalling and apoptosis

Studies performed by Berkowitz's group have demonstrated the role of p38 mitogen-activated protein kinase (p38MAPK) in the pathogenesis of pemphigus. Human keratinocytes treated with PV IgG show a time and dose dependent increase in levels of p38MAPK and heat shock protein 27 (HSP27) proteins involved in regulating cytoskeletal components such as keratin intermediate filaments [186]. Inhibitors of MAPK signalling blocked phosphorylation of HSP27 following PV IgG stimulation of human keratinocytes and importantly prevented keratin filament retraction, an early change evident in acantholysis [186]. Inhibition of p38MAPK in murine and cell culture models of pemphigus vulgaris also prevented blister formation [187],[188]. The same group also recently demonstrated p38MAPK inhibition and prevention of blister formation in a murine model of PF [189]. An open labelled uncontrolled study is currently in progress to determine the safety and efficacy of the oral allosteric p38MAPK inhibitor, KC706 (Kémia, Inc), in refractory PV.

Activation of protein kinase C (PKC) followed by plakoglobin dislocation and subsequent dissociation of desmogleins from desmosomes also appear important in the pathogenesis of pemphigus [190]-[194]. Inhibitors of PKC and plakoglobin/c-myc proto-oncogene axis have been shown to inhibit PV IgG induced blister formation in the neonatal passive transfer murine model of pemphigus vulgaris [195]. It has been demonstrated that p53 knockout mice are protected from PV IgG induced disease [196]. Neonatal mice pre-treated with p53 inhibitor pifithrin-alpha were resistant to both PV and PF IgG mediated blister formation [197].

As shown by the studies of Waschke et al, PV autoantibodies directly block desmoglein-3 transinteraction in contrast to anti-desmoglein antibodies found in PF, which disrupt desmoglein-1 transinteraction via cellular signalling events rather than by direct inhibition [198]-[200]. Hence targeting these signalling proteins in PF may provide a more specific target of therapy as compared to immunosuppressive or biological agents. It remains to be determined whether targeting these signalling proteins results in mediating disease remission in humans. Although they target specific areas of pemphigus pathogenesis, these proteins mediate numerous cellular functions and hence the outcome of early safety studies is eagerly awaited.

11. Elimination of triggering antigens

The elimination or avoidance of an antigen in a genetically susceptible individual may prevent the onset of disease or reduce disease activity. Cessation of offending medications such as penicillamine or captopril results in remission of drug-induced PF [25],[201], [202]. Similarly, patients with endemic pemphigus, who relocate from their native rural endemic environment to a more industrialized area experience clinical and immunologic disease regression [203]. Hence, the clear identification of a triggering environmental antigen such as arthropod protein, microorganism or otherwise, will not only enhance our understanding of disease pathogenesis but also significantly enhance therapies in endemic pemphigus and possibly non-endemic PF [5].

12. Conclusion

PV and PF are debilitating and potentially life-threatening conditions that are therefore important to promptly recognize clinically and then confirm through their characteristic features on histology and direct immunofluorescence. The detection of serum autoantibodies by indirect immunofluorescence or ELISA does not obviate the need for a tissue diagnosis but might be useful is assessing disease severity and activity.

Although, corticosteroids remain the cornerstone of therapy for pemphigus, the morbidity associated with its use restricts its value as a long term treatment option. This is complicated by the fact that steroid-sparing agents are also associated with serious adverse events and there are only few randomized controlled trials demonstrating a beneficial response from the use of these agents. This has been further compounded, until very recently, by the inconsistent parameters of disease activity used in different studies. Azathioprine and mycophenolate mofetil appear to be the most feasible first line adjunctive agents in terms of inducing and

http://dx.doi.org/10.5772/56423

maintaining remission and having a comparatively favourable side effect profile. An enhanced understanding of the pathogenesis of pemphigus has resulted in the implementation of a number of novel agents. These therapies have also been mainly studies through case series reports, are expensive and difficult to access in some centres, and are associated with a number of deleterious side effects. Rituximab, has emerged as the therapy of choice in severe refractory disease and is now being explored as a first line agent. We eagerly await further studies on the effects and safety profiles of more specific agents, especially those targeting signalling molecules involved in the pathogenesis of pemphigus.

We have formulated guidelines on the treatment of pemphigus as suggested by the current level of evidence [204]. Corticosteroids remain the mainstay of treatment and should be initiated at a dose of 0.5 mg /kg of oral prednisone per day and continued at this dose until disease control is obtained. This is defined as the time at which new lesions cease to form and existing lesions begin to heal and in responsive patients, this usually occurs within weeks. At the end of the consolidation phase defined as the point in time where no new lesions have occurred after 2 weeks and 80% of established lesions have healed, the corticosteroid dose is tapered. Unless disease is mild we would recommend adding an adjuvant agent. Either mycophenolate mofetil or azathioprine could be utilized at this stage. For severe or recalcitrant disease rituximab is recommended given the current level of evidence. Other biologic agents, extracorporeal therapies or cytotoxic agents can be considered if rituximab is unavailable or contraindicated.

Author details

Suran L. Fernando[1,2], Jamma Li[1] and Mark Schifter[3,4]

1 Department of Clinical Immunology and Allergy, Royal North Shore Hospital, Sydney, Australia

2 Sydney Medical School – Northern, Sydney University, Sydney, Australia

3 Department of Oral Medicine, Oral Pathology and Special Care Dentistry, Westmead Hospital, (Western) Sydney, Australia

4 Faculty of Dentistry, University of Sydney, Sydney, Australia

References

[1] Chams-Davatchi C, Valikhani M, Daneshpazhooh M, et al. Pemphigus: analysis of 1209 cases. Int J Dermatol 2005;44:470-6.

[2] Uzun S, Durdu M, Akman A, et al. Pemphigus in the Mediterranean region of Turkey: a study of 148 cases. Int J Dermatol 2006;45:523-8.

[3] Krain LS. Pemphigus. Epidemiologic and survival characteristics of 59 patients, 1955-1973. Arch Dermatol 1974;110:862-5.

[4] Aboobaker J, Morar N, Ramdial PK, Hammond MG. Pemphigus in South Africa. Int J Dermatol 2001;40:115-9.

[5] Culton DA, Qian Y, Li N, et al. Advances in pemphigus and its endemic pemphigus foliaceus (Fogo Selvagem) phenotype: a paradigm of human autoimmunity. J Autoimmun 2008;31:311-24.

[6] Abreu-Velez AM, Hashimoto T, Bollag WB, et al. A unique form of endemic pemphigus in northern Colombia. J Am Acad Dermatol 2003;49:599-608.

[7] Bastuji-Garin S, Souissi R, Blum L, et al. Comparative epidemiology of pemphigus in Tunisia and France: unusual incidence of pemphigus foliaceus in young Tunisian women. J Invest Dermatol 1995;104:302-5.

[8] Amagai M, Tsunoda K, Zillikens D, Nagai T, Nishikawa T. The clinical phenotype of pemphigus is defined by the anti-desmoglein autoantibody profile. J Am Acad Dermatol 1999;40:167-70.

[9] Stanley JR, Koulu L, Thivolet C. Distinction between epidermal antigens binding pemphigus vulgaris and pemphigus foliaceus autoantibodies. J Clin Invest 1984;74:313-20.

[10] Koulu L, Kusumi A, Steinberg MS, Klaus-Kovtun V, Stanley JR. Human autoantibodies against a desmosomal core protein in pemphigus foliaceus. J Exp Med 1984;160:1509-18.

[11] Gniadecki R. Desmoglein autoimmunity in the pathogenesis of pemphigus. Autoimmunity 2006;39:541-7.

[12] Anhalt G, Labib K, Vorhees J, Beals T, Diaz L. Induction of pemphigus in neonatal mice by passive transfer of IgG from patients with the disease. N Engl J Med 1982;306:1189-92.

[13] Nishifuji K, Amagai M, Kuwana M, Iwasaki T, Nishukawa T. Detection of antigen-specific B cells in patients with pemphigus vulgaris by enzyme-linked immunospot assay: Requirement of T cell collaboration for autoantibody production. J Invest Dermatol 2000;114:88-94.

[14] Hertl M. Humoral and Cellular Autoimmunity in Autoimmune Bullous Skin Disorders. Int Arch Allergy Immunol 2000;122:91-100.

[15] Bhol K, Ahmed A, Aoki V, Mohimen A, Nagarwalla N, Natarajan K. Correlation of peptide specificity and IgG subclass with pathogenic and non pathogenic autoanti-

bodies in pemphigus vulgaris: A model for autoimmunity. Proc Natl Acad Sci USA 1995;92:5239-43.

[16] Giordano C, Sinha A. Cytokine networks in Pemphigus vulgaris: An integrated viewpoint. Autoimmunity 2012;45:427-39.

[17] Satyam A, Khandpur S, Sharma V, Sharma A. Involvement of Th1/Th2 cytokines in the pathogenesis of autoimmune skin disease - Pemphigus vulgaris. Immunol Invest 2009;38:498-509.

[18] D'Auria L, Bonifati C, Mussi A, et al. Cytokines in the sera of patients with pemphigus vulgaris: interleukin-6 and tumour necrosis factor-alpha levels are significantly increased as compared to healthy subjects and correlate with disease activity. Eur Cytokine Netw 1997;8:383-7.

[19] Lombardi ML, Mercuro O, Ruocco V, et al. Common human leukocyte antigen alleles in pemphigus vulgaris and pemphigus foliaceus Italian patients. J Invest Dermatol 1999;113:107-10.

[20] Loiseau P, Lecleach L, Prost C, et al. HLA class II polymorphism contributes to specify desmoglein derived peptides in pemphigus vulgaris and pemphigus foliaceus. J Autoimmun 2000;15:67-73.

[21] Aoki V, Millikan RC, Rivitti EA, et al. Environmental risk factors in endemic pemphigus foliaceus (fogo selvagem). J Investig Dermatol Symp Proc 2004;9:34-40.

[22] Ribeiro JM, Valenzuela JG, Pham VM, et al. An insight into the sialotranscriptome of Simulium nigrimanum, a black fly associated with fogo selvagem in South America. The American journal of tropical medicine and hygiene 2010;82:1060-75.

[23] Sirois DA, Fatahzadeh M, Roth R, Ettlin D. Diagnostic patterns and delays in pemphigus vulgaris: experience with 99 patients. Arch Dermatol 2000;136:1569-70.

[24] Mourellou O, Chaidemenos GC, Koussidou T, Kapetis E. The treatment of pemphigus vulgaris. Experience with 48 patients seen over an 11-year period. Br J Dermatol 1995;133:83-7.

[25] Kaplan RP, Potter TS, Fox JN. Drug-induced pemphigus related to angiotensin-converting enzyme inhibitors. J Am Acad Dermatol 1992;26:364-6.

[26] Penas PF, Buezo GF, Carvajal I, Dauden E, Lopez A, Diaz LA. D-penicillamine-induced pemphigus foliaceus with autoantibodies to desmoglein-1 in a patient with mixed connective tissue disease. Journal of the American Academy of Dermatology 1997;37:121-3.

[27] Lee CW, Lim JH, Kang HJ. Pemphigus foliaceus induced by rifampicin. The British journal of dermatology 1984;111:619-22.

[28] Ishiko A, Hashimoto T, Shimizu H, et al. Combined features of pemphigus foliaceus and bullous pemphigoid: immunoblot and immunoelectron microscopic studies. Archives of dermatology 1995;131:732-4.

[29] Imamura S, Takigawa M, Ikai K, Yoshinaga H, Yamada M. Pemphigus foliaceus, myasthenia gravis, thymoma and red cell aplasia. A case report and indirect immunofluorescence study on 38 patients with myasthenia gravis. Clinical and experimental dermatology 1978;3:285-91.

[30] Ng PP, Ng SK, Chng HH. Pemphigus foliaceus and oral lichen planus in a patient with systemic lupus erythematosus and thymoma. Clinical and experimental dermatology 1998;23:181-4.

[31] Cowley NC, Neill SM, Staughton RC. Pemphigus foliaceus and non-Hodgkin's lymphoma. International journal of dermatology 1994;33:510-1.

[32] Ota M, Sato-Matsumura KC, Matsumura T, Tsuji Y, Ohkawara A. Pemphigus foliaceus and figurate erythema in a patient with prostate cancer. The British journal of dermatology 2000;142:816-8.

[33] Inaoki M, Kaji K, Furuse S, et al. Pemphigus foliaceus developing after metastasis of cutaneous squamous cell carcinoma to regional lymph nodes. Journal of the American Academy of Dermatology 2001;45:767-70.

[34] Mihai S, Sitaru C. Immunopathology and molecular diagnosis of autoimmune bullous diseases. J Cell Mol Med 2007;11:462-81.

[35] Kneisel A, Hertl M. Autoimmune bullous skin diseases. Part 2: diagnosis and therapy. J Dtsch Dermatol Ges 2011;9:927-47.

[36] Morrison L. Direct immunofluorescence microscopy in the diagnosis of autoimmune bullous dermatoses. Clinics in Dermatology 2001;19:607-13.

[37] Kirtschig G, Wojnarowska F. Autoimmune blistering diseases: an up-date of diagnostic methods and investigations. Clinical and Experimental Dermatology 1994;19:97-112.

[38] Harrist TJ, Mihm MC. Cutaneous immunopathology. The diagnostic use of direct and indirect immunofluorescence techniques in dermatologic disease. Human pathology 1979;10:625-53.

[39] Kanitakis J. Indirect Immunofluorescence Microscopy for the Serological Diagnosis of Autoimmune Blistering Skin Diseases: A Review. Clinics in Dermatology 2001;19:614-21.

[40] Fernando SL, O'Connor KS. Treatment of severe pemphigus foliaceus with rituximab. Med J Aust 2008;189:289-90.

[41] Schmidt E, Dahnrich C, Rosemann A, et al. Novel ELISA systems for antibodies to desmoglein 1 and 3: correlation of disease activity with serum autoantibody levels in individual pemphigus patients. Experimental Dermatology 2010;19:458-63.

[42] Ishii K, Amagal M, Hall R, et al. Characterization of autoantibodies in pemphigus using antigen-specific enzyme linked immunosorbent assays with baculovirus-expressed recombinant desmogleins. J Immunol 1997;159:2010-7.

[43] Schmidt E, Zillikens D. Modern diagnosis of autoimmune blistering skin diseases. Autoimmunity Reviews 2010;10:84-9.

[44] Tampoia M, Giavarina D, Di Giorgio C, Bizzaro N. Diagnostic accuracy of enzyme-linked immunosorbent assays (ELISA) to detect anti-skin autoantibodies in autoimmune blistering skin diseases: A systematic review and meta-analysis. Autoimmunity Reviews 2012;12:121-6.

[45] Harman K, Seed P, Gratian M, Bhogal B, Challacombe S, Black M. The severity of cutaneous and oral pemphigus is related to desmoglein 1 and 3 antibody levels. British Journal of Dermatology 2001;144:775-80.

[46] Hallaji Z, Mortazavi H, Lajevardi V, et al. Serum and salivary desmoglein 1 and 3 enzyme-linked immunosorbent assay in pemphigus vulgaris: correlation with phenotype and severity. J Eur Acad Dermatol Venereol 2010;24:275-80.

[47] Bystryn JC, Steinman NM. The adjuvant therapy of pemphigus. An update. Arch Dermatol 1996;132:203-12.

[48] Castro RM, Roscoe JT, Sampaio SA. Brazilian pemphigus foliaceus. Clin Dermatol 1983;1:22-41.

[49] Diaz LA, Sampaio SA, Rivitti EA, et al. Endemic pemphigus foliaceus (fogo selvagem). I. Clinical features and immunopathology. J Am Acad Dermatol 1989;20:657-69.

[50] Martin LK, Werth V, Villanueva E, Segall J, Murrell DF. Interventions for pemphigus vulgaris and pemphigus foliaceus. Cochrane Database Syst Rev 2009:CD006263.

[51] Murrell DF, Dick S, Ahmed AR, et al. Consensus statement on definitions of disease, end points, and therapeutic response for pemphigus. J Am Acad Dermatol 2008;58:1043-6.

[52] Bystryn JC. Adjuvant therapy of pemphigus. Arch Dermatol 1984;120:941-51.

[53] Ratnam KV, Phay KL, Tan CK. Pemphigus therapy with oral prednisolone regimens. A 5-year study. Int J Dermatol 1990;29:363-7.

[54] Mentink LF, Mackenzie MW, Toth GG, et al. Randomized controlled trial of adjuvant oral dexamethasone pulse therapy in pemphigus vulgaris: PEMPULS trial. Arch Dermatol 2006;142:570-6.

[55] Werth VP. Treatment of pemphigus vulgaris with brief, high-dose intravenous glucocorticoids. Arch Dermatol 1996;132:1435-9.

[56] Femiano F, Gombos F, Scully C. Pemphigus vulgaris with oral involvement: evaluation of two different systemic corticosteroid therapeutic protocols. J Eur Acad Dermatol Venereol 2002;16:353-6.

[57] Mimouni D, Nousari CH, Cummins DL, Kouba DJ, David M, Anhalt GJ. Differences and similarities among expert opinions on the diagnosis and treatment of pemphigus vulgaris. J Am Acad Dermatol 2003;49:1059-62.

[58] Roenigk HH, Jr., Deodhar S. Pemphigus treatment with azathioprine. Clinical and immunologic correlation. Arch Dermatol 1973;107:353-7.

[59] Chams-Davatchi C, Esmaili N, Daneshpazhooh M, et al. Randomized controlled open-label trial of four treatment regimens for pemphigus vulgaris. J Am Acad Dermatol 2007;57:622-8.

[60] Chaidemenos G, Apalla Z, Koussidou T, Papagarifallou I, Ioannides D. High dose oral prednisone vs. prednisone plus azathioprine for the treatment of oral pemphigus: a retrospective, bi-centre, comparative study. J Eur Acad Dermatol Venereol 2011;25:206-10.

[61] Aberer W, Wolff-Schreiner EC, Stingl G, Wolff K. Azathioprine in the treatment of pemphigus vulgaris. A long-term follow-up. J Am Acad Dermatol 1987;16:527-33.

[62] Benoit Corven C, Carvalho P, Prost C, et al. [Treatment of pemphigus vulgaris by azathioprine and low doses of prednisone (Lever scheme)]. Ann Dermatol Venereol 2003;130:13-5.

[63] Krensky AM. Immunosuppressants, Tolerogens, and Immunostimulants. In: Brunton LL, ed. Goodman & Gilman's The Pharmacological Basis of Therapeutics, 11th Edition. 11th ed: McGraw-Hill; 2006.

[64] Beissert S, Werfel T, Frieling U, et al. A comparison of oral methylprednisolone plus azathioprine or mycophenolate mofetil for the treatment of pemphigus. Arch Dermatol 2006;142:1447-54.

[65] Enk AH, Knop J. Mycophenolate is effective in the treatment of pemphigus vulgaris. Arch Dermatol 1999;135:54-6.

[66] Mimouni D, Anhalt GJ, Cummins DL, Kouba DJ, Thorne JE, Nousari HC. Treatment of pemphigus vulgaris and pemphigus foliaceus with mycophenolate mofetil. Arch Dermatol 2003;139:739-42.

[67] Esmaili N, Chams-Davatchi C, Valikhani M, Farshidfar F, Parvaneh N, Tamizifar B. Treatment of pemphigus vulgaris with mycophenolate mofetil as a steroid-sparing agent. Eur J Dermatol 2008;18:159-64.

[68] Enk AH, Knop J. Treatment of pemphigus vulgaris with mycophenolate mofetil. Lancet 1997;350:494.

[69] Powell AM, Albert S, Al Fares S, et al. An evaluation of the usefulness of mycophenolate mofetil in pemphigus. Br J Dermatol 2003;149:138-45.

[70] Orvis AK, Wesson SK, Breza TS, Jr., Church AA, Mitchell CL, Watkins SW. Mycophenolate mofetil in dermatology. J Am Acad Dermatol 2009;60:183-99; quiz 200-2.

[71] Chrysomallis F, Ioannides D, Teknetzis A, Panagiotidou D, Minas A. Treatment of oral pemphigus vulgaris. Int J Dermatol 1994;33:803-7.

[72] Rose E, Wever S, Zilliken D, Linse R, Haustein UF, Brocker EB. Intravenous dexamethasone-cyclophosphamide pulse therapy in comparison with oral methylprednisolone-azathioprine therapy in patients with pemphigus: results of a multicenter prospectively randomized study. J Dtsch Dermatol Ges 2005;3:200-6.

[73] Kaur S, Kanwar AJ. Dexamethasone-cyclophosphamide pulse therapy in pemphigus. Int J Dermatol 1990;29:371-4.

[74] Pasricha JS, Khaitan BK, Raman RS, Chandra M. Dexamethasone-cyclophosphamide pulse therapy for pemphigus. Int J Dermatol 1995;34:875-82.

[75] Fleischli ME, Valek RH, Pandya AG. Pulse intravenous cyclophosphamide therapy in pemphigus. Arch Dermatol 1999;135:57-61.

[76] Ioannides D, Chrysomallis F, Bystryn JC. Ineffectiveness of cyclosporine as an adjuvant to corticosteroids in the treatment of pemphigus. Arch Dermatol 2000;136:868-72.

[77] Mobini N, Padilla T, Jr., Ahmed AR. Long-term remission in selected patients with pemphigus vulgaris treated with cyclosporine. J Am Acad Dermatol 1997;36:264-6.

[78] Werth VP, Fivenson D, Pandya AG, et al. Multicenter randomized, double-blind, placebo-controlled, clinical trial of dapsone as a glucocorticoid-sparing agent in maintenance-phase pemphigus vulgaris. Arch Dermatol 2008;144:25-32.

[79] Heaphy MR, Albrecht J, Werth VP. Dapsone as a glucocorticoid-sparing agent in maintenance-phase pemphigus vulgaris. Arch Dermatol 2005;141:699-702.

[80] Basset N, Guillot B, Michel B, Meynadier J, Guilhou JJ. Dapsone as initial treatment in superficial pemphigus. Report of nine cases. Arch Dermatol 1987;123:783-5.

[81] Gurcan HM, Ahmed AR. Efficacy of dapsone in the treatment of pemphigus and pemphigoid: analysis of current data. Am J Clin Dermatol 2009;10:383-96.

[82] Pfeiffer C, Wozel G. Dapsone and sulfones in dermatology: overview and update. J Am Acad Dermatol 2003;48:308-9.

[83] Smith TJ, Bystryn JC. Methotrexate as an adjuvant treatment for pemphigus vulgaris. Arch Dermatol 1999;135:1275-6.

[84] Mashkilleyson N, Mashkilleyson AL. Mucous membrane manifestations of pemphigus vulgaris. A 25-year survey of 185 patients treated with corticosteroids or with combination of corticosteroids with methotrexate or heparin. Acta Derm Venereol 1988;68:413-21.

[85] Gurcan HM, Ahmed AR. Analysis of current data on the use of methotrexate in the treatment of pemphigus and pemphigoid. Br J Dermatol 2009;161:723-31.

[86] Auad A, Auad T, Auad. A., P. A. Coadjuvant therapy for the treatment of South American pemphigus foliaceus with auraofin, A double-blind study.. Anais Brasileiros de Dermatologia 1986;61:131-4.

[87] Penneys NS, Eaglstein WH, Frost P. Management of pemphigus with gold compounds: a long-term follow-up report. Arch Dermatol 1976;112:185-7.

[88] Poulin Y, Perry HO, Muller SA. Pemphigus vulgaris: results of treatment with gold as a steroid-sparing agent in a series of thirteen patients. J Am Acad Dermatol 1984;11:851-7.

[89] Pandya AG, Dyke C. Treatment of pemphigus with gold. Arch Dermatol 1998;134:1104-7.

[90] Lange D, Meiss F, Fiedler E, Treiber K, Marsch WC, Fischer M. [Gold. Effective therapy for mucosal lesions of pemphigus vulgaris]. Der Hautarzt; Zeitschrift fur Dermatologie, Venerologie, und verwandte Gebiete 2007;58:142-5.

[91] Gaspar ZS, Walkden V, Wojnarowska F. Minocycline is a useful adjuvant therapy for pemphigus. Australas J Dermatol 1996;37:93-5.

[92] Alpsoy E, Yilmaz E, Basaran E, Yazar S, Cetin L. Is the combination of tetracycline and nicotinamide therapy alone effective in pemphigus? Arch Dermatol 1995;131:1339-40.

[93] Calebotta A, Saenz AM, Gonzalez F, Carvalho M, Castillo R. Pemphigus vulgaris: benefits of tetracycline as adjuvant therapy in a series of thirteen patients. Int J Dermatol 1999;38:217-21.

[94] Tabrizi MN, Chams-Davatchi C, Esmaeeli N, et al. Accelerating effects of epidermal growth factor on skin lesions of pemphigus vulgaris: a double-blind, randomized, controlled trial. J Eur Acad Dermatol Venereol 2007;21:79-84.

[95] Dumas V, Roujeau JC, Wolkenstein P, Revuz J, Cosnes A. The treatment of mild pemphigus vulgaris and pemphigus foliaceus with a topical corticosteroid. Br J Dermatol 1999;140:1127-9.

[96] Nghiem P, Pearson G, Langley RG. Tacrolimus and pimecrolimus: from clever prokaryotes to inhibiting calcineurin and treating atopic dermatitis. J Am Acad Dermatol 2002;46:228-41.

[97] Hall VC, Liesegang TJ, Kostick DA, Lookingbill DP. Ocular mucous membrane pemphigoid and ocular pemphigus vulgaris treated topically with tacrolimus ointment. Arch Dermatol 2003;139:1083-4.

[98] Termeer CC, Technau K, Augustin M, Simon JC. Topical tacrolimus (protopic) for the treatment of a localized pemphigus foliaceus. J Eur Acad Dermatol Venereol 2004;18:636-7.

[99] Cassano N, Coviello C, Scoppio BM, Miracapillo A, Vena GA. Recalcitrant lesions of pemphigus foliaceous at a surgical site: successful treatment with tacrolimus 0.1% ointment. Eur J Dermatol 2006;16:443-4.

[100] Iraji F, Asilian A, Siadat AH. Pimecrolimus 1% cream in the treatment of cutaneous lesions of pemphigus vulgaris: a double-blind, placebo-controlled clinical trial. Journal of drugs in dermatology : JDD 2010;9:684-6.

[101] Browning JL. B cells move to centre stage: novel opportunities for autoimmune disease treatment. Nat Rev Drug Discov 2006;5:564-76.

[102] Edwards JC, Cambridge G. Prospects for B-cell-targeted therapy in autoimmune disease. Rheumatology (Oxford) 2005;44:151-6.

[103] Eming R, Nagel A, Wolff-Franke S, Podstawa E, Debus D, Hertl M. Rituximab exerts a dual effect in pemphigus vulgaris. J Invest Dermatol 2008;128:2850-8.

[104] Cellerai C, Harari A, Vallelian F, Boyman O, Pantaleo G. Functional and phenotypic characterization of tetanus toxoid-specific human CD4+ T cells following re-immunization. Eur J Immunol 2007;37:1129-38.

[105] Herrmann G, Hunzelmann N, Engert A. Treatment of pemphigus vulgaris with anti-CD20 monoclonal antibody (rituximab). Br J Dermatol 2003;148:602-3.

[106] Goebeler M, Herzog S, Brocker EB, Zillikens D. Rapid response of treatment-resistant pemphigus foliaceus to the anti-CD20 antibody rituximab. Br J Dermatol 2003;149:899-901.

[107] Dupuy A, Viguier M, Bedane C, et al. Treatment of refractory pemphigus vulgaris with rituximab (anti-CD20 monoclonal antibody). Arch Dermatol 2004;140:91-6.

[108] Espana A, Fernandez-Galar M, Lloret P, Sanchez-Ibarrola A, Panizo C. Long-term complete remission of severe pemphigus vulgaris with monoclonal anti-CD20 antibody therapy and immunophenotype correlations. J Am Acad Dermatol 2004;50:974-6.

[109] Morrison LH. Therapy of refractory pemphigus vulgaris with monoclonal anti-CD20 antibody (rituximab). J Am Acad Dermatol 2004;51:817-9.

[110] Wenzel J, Bauer R, Bieber T, Tuting T. Successful rituximab treatment of severe pemphigus vulgaris resistant to multiple immunosuppressants. Acta Derm Venereol 2005;85:185-6.

[111] Schmidt E, Herzog S, Brocker EB, Zillikens D, Goebeler M. Long-standing remission of recalcitrant juvenile pemphigus vulgaris after adjuvant therapy with rituximab. Br J Dermatol 2005;153:449-51.

[112] Arin MJ, Engert A, Krieg T, Hunzelmann N. Anti-CD20 monoclonal antibody (rituximab) in the treatment of pemphigus. Br J Dermatol 2005;153:620-5.

[113] Kong HH, Prose NS, Ware RE, Hall RP, 3rd. Successful treatment of refractory childhood pemphgus vulgaris with anti-CD20 monoclonal antibody (rituximab). Pediatr Dermatol 2005;22:461-4.

[114] El Tal AK, Posner MR, Spigelman Z, Ahmed AR. Rituximab: a monoclonal antibody to CD20 used in the treatment of pemphigus vulgaris. J Am Acad Dermatol 2006;55:449-59.

[115] Serrao VV, Martins A, Paris FR, Lopes MP. Successful treatment of recalcitrant pemphigus foliaceus with rituximab. J Eur Acad Dermatol Venereol 2008;22:768-70.

[116] Cianchini G, Lupi F, Masini C, Corona R, Puddu P, De Pita O. Therapy with rituximab for autoimmune pemphigus: results from a single-center observational study on 42 cases with long-term follow-up. Journal of the American Academy of Dermatology 2012;67:617-22.

[117] Joly P, Mouquet H, Roujeau JC, et al. A single cycle of rituximab for the treatment of severe pemphigus. N Engl J Med 2007;357:545-52.

[118] Cianchini G, Corona R, Frezzolini A, Ruffelli M, Didona B, Puddu P. Treatment of severe pemphigus with rituximab: report of 12 cases and a review of the literature. Arch Dermatol 2007;143:1033-8.

[119] Ahmed AR, Spigelman Z, Cavacini LA, Posner MR. Treatment of pemphigus vulgaris with rituximab and intravenous immune globulin. N Engl J Med 2006;355:1772-9.

[120] Kasperkiewicz M, Shimanovich I, Meier M, et al. Treatment of severe pemphigus with a combination of immunoadsorption, rituximab, pulsed dexamethasone and azathioprine/mycophenolate mofetil: a pilot study of 23 patients. The British journal of dermatology 2012;166:154-60.

[121] Horvath B, Huizinga J, Pas HH, Mulder AB, Jonkman MF. Low-dose rituximab is effective in pemphigus. The British journal of dermatology 2012;166:405-12.

[122] Mouquet H, Musette P, Gougeon ML, et al. B-cell depletion immunotherapy in pemphigus: effects on cellular and humoral immune responses. J Invest Dermatol 2008;128:2859-69.

[123] Schmidt E, Brocker EB, Goebeler M. Rituximab in treatment-resistant autoimmune blistering skin disorders. Clin Rev Allergy Immunol 2008;34:56-64.

[124] Molloy ES, Calabrese LH. Progressive multifocal leukoencephalopathy associated with immunosuppressive therapy in rheumatic diseases: evolving role of biologic therapies. Arthritis and rheumatism 2012;64:3043-51.

[125] Padgett BL, Walker DL, ZuRhein GM, Eckroade RJ, Dessel BH. Cultivation of papova-like virus from human brain with progressive multifocal leucoencephalopathy. Lancet 1971;1:1257-60.

[126] Cohen Y, Solal-Celigny P, Polliack A. Rituximab therapy for follicular lymphoma: a comprehensive review of its efficacy as primary treatment, treatment for relapsed disease, re-treatment and maintenance. Haematologica 2003;88:811-23.

[127] Hertl M, Eming R, Borradori L. Rituximab (anti-CD20 monoclonal antibody)--ultimate or first choice in pemphigus? Dermatology 2007;214:275-7.

[128] Feliciani C, Toto P, Amerio P, et al. In vitro and in vivo expression of interleukin-1alpha and tumor necrosis factor-alpha mRNA in pemphigus vulgaris: interleukin-1alpha and tumor necrosis factor-alpha are involved in acantholysis. J Invest Dermatol 2000;114:71-7.

[129] Lopez-Robles E, Avalos-Diaz E, Vega-Memije E, et al. TNFalpha and IL-6 are mediators in the blistering process of pemphigus. Int J Dermatol 2001;40:185-8.

[130] Berookhim B, Fischer HD, Weinberg JM. Treatment of recalcitrant pemphigus vulgaris with the tumor necrosis factor alpha antagonist etanercept. Cutis 2004;74:245-7.

[131] Lin MH, Hsu CK, Lee JY. Successful treatment of recalcitrant pemphigus vulgaris and pemphigus vegetans with etanercept and carbon dioxide laser. Arch Dermatol 2005;141:680-2.

[132] Gubinelli E, Bergamo F, Didona B, Annessi G, Atzori F, Raskovic D. Pemphigus foliaceus treated with etanercept. J Am Acad Dermatol 2006;55:1107-8.

[133] Shetty A, Marcum CB, Glass LF, Carter JD. Successful treatment of pemphigus vulgaris with etanercept in four patients. Journal of drugs in dermatology : JDD 2009;8:940-3.

[134] Jacobi A, Shuler G, Hertl M. Rapid control of therapy-refractory pemphigus vulgaris by treatment with the tumour necrosis factor-alpha inhibitor infliximab. Br J Dermatol 2005;153:448-9.

[135] Pardo J, Mercader P, Mahiques L, Sanchez-Carazo JL, Oliver V, Fortea JM. Infliximab in the management of severe pemphigus vulgaris. Br J Dermatol 2005;153:222-3.

[136] Howell SM, Bessinger GT, Altman CE, Belnap CM. Rapid response of IgA pemphigus of the subcorneal pustular dermatosis subtype to treatment with adalimumab and mycophenolate mofetil. J Am Acad Dermatol 2005;53:541-3.

[137] Jolles S, Sewell WA, Misbah SA. Clinical uses of intravenous immunoglobulin. Clin Exp Immunol 2005;142:1-11.

[138] Kazatchkine MD, Kaveri SV. Immunomodulation of autoimmune and inflammatory diseases with intravenous immune globulin. N Engl J Med 2001;345:747-55.

[139] Zhu KY, Feferman T, Maiti PK, Souroujon MC, Fuchs S. Intravenous immunoglobulin suppresses experimental myasthenia gravis: immunological mechanisms. J Neuroimmunol 2006;176:187-97.

[140] Arredondo J, Chernyavsky AI, Karaouni A, Grando SA. Novel mechanisms of target cell death and survival and of therapeutic action of IVIg in Pemphigus. Am J Pathol 2005;167:1531-44.

[141] Bystryn JC, Jiao D. IVIg selectively and rapidly decreases circulating pathogenic autoantibodies in pemphigus vulgaris. Autoimmunity 2006;39:601-7.

[142] Green MG, Bystryn JC. Effect of intravenous immunoglobulin therapy on serum levels of IgG1 and IgG4 antidesmoglein 1 and antidesmoglein 3 antibodies in pemphigus vulgaris. Arch Dermatol 2008;144:1621-4.

[143] Sami N, Bhol KC, Ahmed AR. Influence of IVIg therapy on autoantibody titers to desmoglein 1 in patients with pemphigus foliaceus. Clin Immunol 2002;105:192-8.

[144] Li N, Zhao M, Hilario-Vargas J, et al. Complete FcRn dependence for intravenous Ig therapy in autoimmune skin blistering diseases. J Clin Invest 2005;115:3440-50.

[145] Ahmed AR. Intravenous immunoglobulin therapy in the treatment of patients with pemphigus vulgaris unresponsive to conventional immunosuppressive treatment. J Am Acad Dermatol 2001;45:679-90.

[146] Bystryn JC, Jiao D, Natow S. Treatment of pemphigus with intravenous immunoglobulin. J Am Acad Dermatol 2002;47:358-63.

[147] Sami N, Qureshi A, Ruocco E, Ahmed AR. Corticosteroid-sparing effect of intravenous immunoglobulin therapy in patients with pemphigus vulgaris. Arch Dermatol 2002;138:1158-62.

[148] Baum S, Scope A, Barzilai A, Azizi E, Trau H. The role of IVIg treatment in severe pemphigus vulgaris. J Eur Acad Dermatol Venereol 2006;20:548-52.

[149] Sami N, Qureshi A, Ahmed AR. Steroid sparing effect of intravenous immunoglobulin therapy in patients with pemphigus foliaceus. Eur J Dermatol 2002;12:174-8.

[150] Ahmed AR, Sami N. Intravenous immunoglobulin therapy for patients with pemphigus foliaceus unresponsive to conventional therapy. J Am Acad Dermatol 2002;46:42-9.

[151] Wetter DA, Davis MD, Yiannias JA, et al. Effectiveness of intravenous immunoglobulin therapy for skin disease other than toxic epidermal necrolysis: a retrospective review of Mayo Clinic experience. Mayo Clin Proc 2005;80:41-7.

[152] Segura S, Iranzo P, Martinez-de Pablo I, et al. High-dose intravenous immunoglobulins for the treatment of autoimmune mucocutaneous blistering diseases: evaluation of its use in 19 cases. J Am Acad Dermatol 2007;56:960-7.

[153] Amagai M, Ikeda S, Shimizu H, et al. A randomized double-blind trial of intravenous immunoglobulin for pemphigus. J Am Acad Dermatol 2009;60:595-603.

[154] Bystryn JC, Schenkein I, Uhr JW. A model for regulation of antibody synthesis by serum antibody. Prog Immunol 1971;1:627-36.

[155] Guillaume JC, Roujeau JC, Morel P, et al. Controlled study of plasma exchange in pemphigus. Arch Dermatol 1988;124:1659-63.

[156] Nagasaka T, Fujii Y, Ishida A, et al. Evaluating efficacy of plasmapheresis for patients with pemphigus using desmoglein enzyme-linked immunosorbent assay. Br J Dermatol 2008;158:685-90.

[157] Roujeau JC, Andre C, Joneau Fabre M, et al. Plasma exchange in pemphigus. Uncontrolled study of ten patients. Arch Dermatol 1983;119:215-21.

[158] Ruocco V, Astarita C, Pisani M. Plasmapheresis as an alternative or adjunctive therapy in problem cases of pemphigus. Dermatologica 1984;168:219-23.

[159] Blaszczyk M, Chorzelski TP, Jablonska S, Daszynski J, Beutner EH. Indications for future studies on the treatment of pemphigus with plasmapheresis. Arch Dermatol 1989;125:843-4.

[160] Tan-Lim R, Bystryn JC. Effect of plasmapheresis therapy on circulating levels of pemphigus antibodies. J Am Acad Dermatol 1990;22:35-40.

[161] Sondergaard K, Carstens J, Zachariae H. The steroid-sparing effect of long-term plasmapheresis in pemphigus: An update. Ther Apher 1997;1:155-8.

[162] Eming R, Hertl M. Immunoadsorption in pemphigus. Autoimmunity 2006;39:609-16.

[163] Ogata K, Yasuda K, Matsushita M, Kodama H. Successful treatment of adolescent pemphigus vulgaris by immunoadsorption method. J Dermatol 1999;26:236-9.

[164] Schmidt E, Klinker E, Opitz A, et al. Protein A immunoadsorption: a novel and effective adjuvant treatment of severe pemphigus. Br J Dermatol 2003;148:1222-9.

[165] Luftl M, Stauber A, Mainka A, Klingel R, Schuler G, Hertl M. Successful removal of pathogenic autoantibodies in pemphigus by immunoadsorption with a tryptophan-linked polyvinylalcohol adsorber. Br J Dermatol 2003;149:598-605.

[166] Frost N, Messer G, Fierlbeck G, Risler T, Lytton SD. Treatment of pemphigus vulgaris with protein A immunoadsorption: case report of long-term history showing favorable outcome. Ann N Y Acad Sci 2005;1051:591-6.

[167] Shimanovich I, Herzog S, Schmidt E, et al. Improved protocol for treatment of pemphigus vulgaris with protein A immunoadsorption. Clin Exp Dermatol 2006;31:768-74.

[168] Shimanovich I, Nitschke M, Rose C, Grabbe J, Zillikens D. Treatment of severe pemphigus with protein A immunoadsorption, rituximab and intravenous immunoglobulins. Br J Dermatol 2008;158:382-8.

[169] Pfutze M, Eming R, Kneisel A, Kuhlmann U, Hoyer J, Hertl M. Clinical and immunological follow-up of pemphigus patients on adjuvant treatment with immunoadsorption or rituximab. Dermatology 2009;218:237-45.

[170] Hivelin M, Siemionow M, Grimbert P, Lantieri L. Extracorporeal photopheresis: From solid organs to face transplantation. Transpl Immunol 2009.

[171] Voll RE, Herrmann M, Roth EA, Stach C, Kalden JR, Girkontaite I. Immunosuppressive effects of apoptotic cells. Nature 1997;390:350-1.

[172] Wolf R, Matz H, Ruocco E, Ruocco V. The putative role of apoptosis in the induction of pemphigus. Med Hypotheses 2005;64:44-5.

[173] Yeh SW, Sami N, Ahmed RA. Treatment of pemphigus vulgaris: current and emerging options. Am J Clin Dermatol 2005;6:327-42.

[174] Rook AH, Jegasothy BV, Heald P, et al. Extracorporeal photochemotherapy for drug-resistant pemphigus vulgaris. Ann Intern Med 1990;112:303-5.

[175] Liang G, Nahass G, Kerdel FA. Pemphigus vulgaris treated with photopheresis. J Am Acad Dermatol 1992;26:779-80.

[176] Gollnick HP, Owsianowski M, Taube KM, Orfanos CE. Unresponsive severe generalized pemphigus vulgaris successfully controlled by extracorporeal photopheresis. J Am Acad Dermatol 1993;28:122-4.

[177] Wollina U, Lange D, Looks A. Short-time extracorporeal photochemotherapy in the treatment of drug-resistant autoimmune bullous diseases. Dermatology 1999;198:140-4.

[178] Nguyen VT, Arredondo J, Chernyavsky AI, Pittelkow MR, Kitajima Y, Grando SA. Pemphigus vulgaris acantholysis ameliorated by cholinergic agonists. Arch Dermatol 2004;140:327-34.

[179] Grando SA, Dahl, M.V. Activation of keratinocyte muscarinic acetylcholine receptors reverses pemphigus acantholysis. J Eur Acad Dermatol Venereol 1993;2:72-86.

[180] Nguyen VT, Ndoye A, Grando SA. Novel human alpha9 acetylcholine receptor regulating keratinocyte adhesion is targeted by Pemphigus vulgaris autoimmunity. Am J Pathol 2000;157:1377-91.

[181] Nguyen VT, Ndoye A, Grando SA. Pemphigus vulgaris antibody identifies pemphaxin. A novel keratinocyte annexin-like molecule binding acetylcholine. J Biol Chem 2000;275:29466-76.

[182] Nguyen VT, Ndoye A, Shultz LD, Pittelkow MR, Grando SA. Antibodies against keratinocyte antigens other than desmogleins 1 and 3 can induce pemphigus vulgaris-like lesions. J Clin Invest 2000;106:1467-79.

[183] Grando SA. New approaches to the treatment of pemphigus. J Investig Dermatol Symp Proc 2004;9:84-91.

[184] Iraji F, Yoosefi A. Healing effect of Pilocarpine gel 4% on skin lesions of pemphigus vulgaris. Int J Dermatol 2006;45:743-6.

[185] Anhalt GJ, Werth VP, Strober B. An open-label phase I clinical study to assess the safety of PI-0824 in patients with pemphigus vulgaris. J Invest Dermatol 2005;125:1088.

[186] Berkowitz P, Hu P, Liu Z, et al. Desmosome signaling. Inhibition of p38MAPK prevents pemphigus vulgaris IgG-induced cytoskeleton reorganization. J Biol Chem 2005;280:23778-84.

[187] Berkowitz P, Hu P, Warren S, Liu Z, Diaz LA, Rubenstein DS. p38MAPK inhibition prevents disease in pemphigus vulgaris mice. Proc Natl Acad Sci U S A 2006;103:12855-60.

[188] Berkowitz P, Diaz LA, Hall RP, Rubenstein DS. Induction of p38MAPK and HSP27 phosphorylation in pemphigus patient skin. J Invest Dermatol 2008;128:738-40.

[189] Berkowitz P, Chua M, Liu Z, Diaz LA, Rubenstein DS. Autoantibodies in the autoimmune disease pemphigus foliaceus induce blistering via p38 mitogen-activated protein kinase-dependent signaling in the skin. Am J Pathol 2008;173:1628-36.

[190] Kitajima Y, Aoyama Y, Seishima M. Transmembrane signaling for adhesive regulation of desmosomes and hemidesmosomes, and for cell-cell datachment induced by pemphigus IgG in cultured keratinocytes: involvement of protein kinase C. J Investig Dermatol Symp Proc 1999;4:137-44.

[191] Aoyama Y, Kitajima Y. Pemphigus vulgaris-IgG causes a rapid depletion of desmoglein 3 (Dsg3) from the Triton X-100 soluble pools, leading to the formation of Dsg3-depleted desmosomes in a human squamous carcinoma cell line, DJM-1 cells. J Invest Dermatol 1999;112:67-71.

[192] Aoyama Y, Owada MK, Kitajima Y. A pathogenic autoantibody, pemphigus vulgaris-IgG, induces phosphorylation of desmoglein 3, and its dissociation from plakoglobin in cultured keratinocytes. Eur J Immunol 1999;29:2233-40.

[193] Caldelari R, de Bruin A, Baumann D, et al. A central role for the armadillo protein plakoglobin in the autoimmune disease pemphigus vulgaris. J Cell Biol 2001;153:823-34.

[194] Lo Muzio L, Pannone G, Staibano S, et al. A possible role of catenin dyslocalization in pemphigus vulgaris pathogenesis. J Cutan Pathol 2001;28:460-9.

[195] Williamson L, Raess NA, Caldelari R, et al. Pemphigus vulgaris identifies plakoglobin as key suppressor of c-Myc in the skin. EMBO J 2006;25:3298-309.

[196] Li N, Liu, Z., Park, M., Diaz, L.A. p53-knockout mice are resistant to the induction of skin blisters and acantholysis by pemphigus autoantibodies. In: Annual meeting SID; 2008; Japan; 2008.

[197] Li N, Liu, Z., Wang, J., Warren, S.J.P., Diaz, L.A. Inhibition of experimental pemphigus by the p53 inhibitor pifithrin-alpha. J Invest Dermatol 2007;127:Abstract 64.

[198] Heupel WM, Zillikens D, Drenckhahn D, Waschke J. Pemphigus vulgaris IgG directly inhibit desmoglein 3-mediated transinteraction. J Immunol 2008;181:1825-34.

[199] Heupel WM, Muller T, Efthymiadis A, Schmidt E, Drenckhahn D, Waschke J. Peptides Targeting the Desmoglein 3 Adhesive Interface Prevent Autoantibody-induced Acantholysis in Pemphigus. J Biol Chem 2009;284:8589-95.

[200] Waschke J, Bruggeman P, Baumgartner W, Zillikens D, Drenckhahn D. Pemphigus foliaceus IgG causes dissociation of desmoglein 1-containing junctions without blocking desmoglein 1 transinteraction. J Clin Invest 2005;115:3157-65.

[201] Bialy-Golan A, Brenner S. Penicillamine-induced bullous dermatoses. J Am Acad Dermatol 1996;35:732-42.

[202] Nagao K, Tanikawa A, Yamamoto N, Amagai M. Decline of anti-desmoglein 1 IgG ELISA scores by withdrawal of D-penicillamine in drug-induced pemphigus foliaceus. Clin Exp Dermatol 2005;30:43-5.

[203] Diaz LA, Sampaio SA, Rivitti EA, et al. Endemic pemphigus foliaceus (Fogo Selvagem): II. Current and historic epidemiologic studies. J Invest Dermatol 1989;92:4-12.

[204] Fernando SL, Broadfoot AJ. Treatment options for pemphigus foliaceus. Giornale italiano di dermatologia e venereologia : organo ufficiale, Societa italiana di dermatologia e sifilografia 2009;144:363-77.

Chapter 6

Oral Lichen Planus

Mark Schifter, Suran L. Fernando and Jamma Li

Additional information is available at the end of the chapter

http://dx.doi.org/10.5772/56482

1. Introduction

Lichen planus is a chronic systemic disease of established immune-mediated pathogenesis. [1] It most commonly, protractedly and persistently, involves the mucosa of the oral cavity, but it can involve other sites, namely the skin, the scalp (with inflammation around and affecting the hair follicles) resulting in alopecia), the nails as well as the genital area - the vulval and vaginal mucosa, and the glans penis. Other sites of involvement that are far less frequently described include the oesophagus and conjunctiva. There are seven recognized oral presentations of lichen planus: (1) reticular, (2) papular, and (3) plaque-form and the (4) atrophic, (5) ulcerative (erosive) and rare (6) vesiculo-bullous form [2] and (7) desquamative gingivitis, this latter term is a clinical descriptor, used to describe inflammation, with a mix of erythema, erosion and/or ulceration of the gingival tissues and the immediately adjacent alveolar mucosa, not incited by the presence of dental bacterial plaque. These latter four forms of OLP can be associated with significant discomfort requiring either topical and/or systemic immunosuppressive therapy.

The cause(s) of the various oral lichenoid lesions, ranging from idiopathic oral lichen planus (OLP) to the "contact" lesion, is not understood, but all the lesions are characterized histologically by a typical "lichenoid tissue reaction" featuring (1) a bandlike lymphohistiocytic infiltrate that fills the lamina propria; and (2) liquefactive degeneration of the basal keratinocytes. [3] These reactions may be the result of several diverse possible triggers, but all culminate in a common pathologic process, that of T-lymphocyte directed, immune mediated, damage to the oral epithelial basal cells.[1, 2]

2. Historical overview

Ferdinand Ritter von Hebra (1816-1880), famed dermatologist and co-founder of the renowned Vienna School of Dermatology, is credited with the first scientific description of the skin disease, he termed leichen ruber planus (in 1860). [4] But it was the famed British Dermatologist, Erasmus Wilson (1809-1884), who originally used the term lichen planus in his publication in 1869, noting the disorder in a group of 50 patients. [5] Lichen planus obtained its name because of the lacy white lines that bear a close resemblance to the symbiont, lichen, a composite organism consisting of a fungus (the mycobiont) and a photosynthetic partner (the photobiont or phycobiont, usually, a green algae) living together in a symbiotic relationship, seen growing on rocks (Figure 1). However, Ferdinand Ritter von Hebra used the term "lichen" to denote skin lesions which are exclusively nodular, that is characterised by a macular-papular skin eruption, hence, terms such as lichen pilaris (better known as Keratosis pilaris), and lichen nitidus are still used for other skin diseases, whose appearance differs markedly from that of lichen planus. [4] Heinrich Köbner (1838–1904) described the phenomenon that bears his name in 1872, at a meeting of the Silesian Society for National Culture. Four years later (1876) he published a paper describing his original patient describing the development of isomorphic pathologic lesions in response to trauma in previously uninvolved sites of patients with skin diseases, most often seen in patients with psoriasis, but also in eczema and lichen planus. [6] These new lesions are clinically and histopathologically identical to those in the diseased skin and/or mucosa. Louis Frédéric Wickham (1861-1913) is acknowledged as the first to describe the characteristic, fine, white or grey lines known as Wickham's striae (striae is derived from Latin for groove) or dots seen on the top of the pruritic papular rash of lichen planus of the skin, and also seen with OLP. [7] In 1910 François Henri Hallopeau reported the first case of OLP-related oral carcinoma. [8]

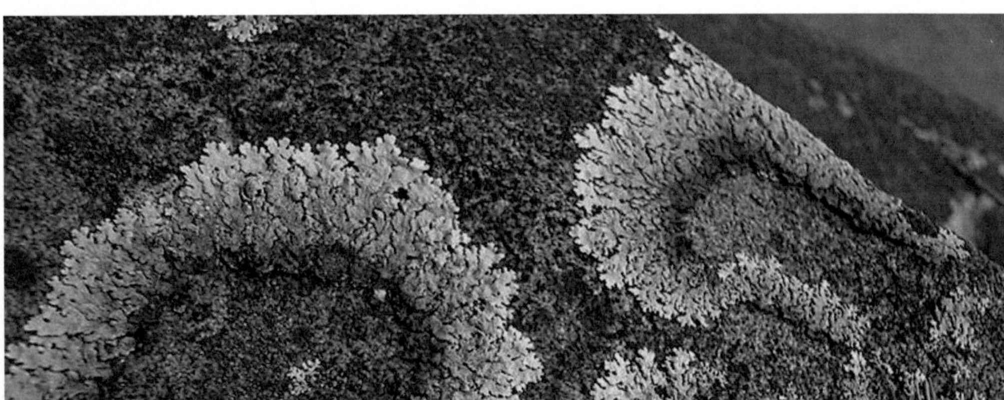

Figure 1. Foliose lichens growing on rock

2.1. Epidemiology

OLP is a common condition, with a prevalence of between 0.5-2.2% of the population. [1, 9] However, a recent review of epidemiological studies specific to OLP, found only one study as being the most useful, being the most free of error and bias and so, is regarded as the most reliable estimation of population prevalence of OLP, at least in European populations with a reported prevalence of 1.27%. [10, 11] However, OLP most frequently presents in women, aged 40 years and above, by a ratio of approximately 3:1 to 3:2 compared with men, of the same age.

2.2. Pathogenesis

The oral mucosa appears to have a limited immunological repertoire, predominantly a lichenoid-type reaction. This is characterised by delayed-type IV hypersensitivity reaction, dominated by cytotoxic $CD8^+$ T-lymphocyte induced apoptosis of the basal keratinocytes, being the final common immunopathological pathway due to variety of insults, such as the development of autoantibodies against self-antigens, interaction with allergens, such as various drugs or dental materials, viruses, namely Hepatitis C (HCV), trauma (mechanical and chemical) and even stress. [12] However, the specifics, including the precise triggering factors, remain unknown and elusive.

The mechanisms involved in the aetio-pathogenesis of OLP are multifactorial and likely to be synergistic:

1. antigen-specific cell-mediated immune response
2. loss of tolerance evidenced by the development of autoantibodies against self-antigens and the promotion of autoimmunity
3. role of the humoral immune response
4. non-specific immune mechanisms; and
5. genetic factors.

3. Antigen-specific cell-mediated immune response

The antigen that serves as the trigger and/or driver of the immune responses seen in OLP is unknown. It is likely, in the majority of cases, to be an endogenous peptide, a protein sequence innate to the basal keratinocyte; therefore, OLP can be characterised as an auto-immune condition. It is also likely that supposed exogenous triggers for OLP, such as dental materials, certain drugs, viruses and even trauma serve to expose such self-antigens, or, alter the normal innate peptide sequences so that they are perceived by the immune-surveillance cells and system as being "non-self, that is "foreign". The immune responses to this, as yet, unidentified antigen develops in three stages: (1) T-cell migration into the epithelium, (2) T-cell activation, followed by (3) induction of basal keratinocyte apoptosis. [12]

T-Cell Migration into the Epithelium: Two hypotheses have been proposed to explain this occurrence. The "chance encounter" hypothesis suggests that normally circulating, antigen-specific CD8+ cytotoxic T-cells enter the epithelium for routine surveillance and by chance encounter the putative antigen when it is present in the epithelium. Alternatively, the keratinocytes direct the CD8+ cytotoxic T-cells to migrate into the epithelium by the release of cytokines that allow the lymphocytes to "home-in" on the antigen-bearing basal keratinocyte, the so called "directed migration" hypothesis. [12, 13]

T-cell Activation: The lymphocytic infiltration that characterises the OLP lesion histologically, is comprised predominantly of T-cells. The majority of the T-cells in proximity to the damaged and dying basal keratinocytes and within the epithelial layers are overwhelmingly activated cytotoxic CD8^{+} T-cells. [14] Cytotoxic CD8+ T-cells binding of antigen on the MHC Class I site of keratinocytes releases cytokines that attract other lymphocytes and immune-cells into the site of the developing OLP lesion. The cytotoxic CD8+ T-cells are also activated by the CD4^{+} helper cells found in the lamina propria. In OLP lesions, helper CD4+ T cells may be activated by antigen associated with Class II MHC presented by the professional antigen-presenting cells, the Langerhans cells, or, by the keratinocytes themselves, which are induced to present antigens on their Class II MHC sites. Langerhans cells are not only increased in number in OLP lesions but also have up-regulated Class II MHC expression. [14] Interleukin-12 (IL-12) is secreted by Class II MHC expressing Langerhans cells and keratinocytes which in turn promotes CD4+ T-cell secretion of interleukin-2 (IL-2) and interferon-γ (IFN- γ). These cytokines (IL-12, IL-2 and IFN- γ) and probably others, together with the presentation of an antigen associated with MHC class I on basal keratinocytes, promote cytotoxic CD8+ T-cell induction of keratinocytes apoptosis. So it would appear that within the OLP lesion there is a cycle of self-inducing and self-perpetuating T-lymphocyte activation.

Basal Keratinocyte Apoptosis: The apoptosis of the basal keratinocytes that characterises all forms of lichen planus, appears to be mediated predominantly by particularly active, cytotoxic CD8+ T-cells. [14] In one study of testing the reactivity of lesional versus non-lesional T-cell clones from LP patients against lesional and non-lesional autologous keratinocytes, the lesional T-cells lines derived from patients with LP were significantly more active and cytotoxic against autologous lesional keratinocytes than the T-cell lines obtained from clinically normal skin. [14] In this same study, it was also shown that the most cytotoxic T-cell clones were CD8^{+} and the least cytotoxic clones, were CD4^{+}. [15] However, in this same study, the cytotoxicity of some of these activated CD8^{+} T-cell clones was shown to be partially inhibited by anti-MHC class I monoclonal antibody (Dako clone W6/32). This antibody targets a monomorphic epitope on the 45 kDa polypeptide products of the HLA-A, B and C loci. [16] These findings indicated that the apoptosis of the basal keratinocytes so characteristic of LP (and OLP) is induced by the cytotoxic CD8+ T-lymphocytes activated by a putative basal keratinocyte antigen associated with the MHC Class I.

The induction of keratinocytes apoptosis by CD8+ T-cells can occur by three established pathways: Firstly, secretion by T-cells of tumour necrosis factor-α (TNF-α), which binds TNF-α receptor 1 on the keratinocytes surface [16] ; secondly, expression on the T-cell surface of CD95L (Fas ligand), which binds CD95 (Fas) on the keratinocytes surface. Fas ligand (FasL or

http://dx.doi.org/10.5772/56482

CD95L) is a type-II transmembrane protein that belongs to the TNF family that on binding with its receptor induces apoptosis in the target cell. [17] Fas-induced apoptosis by the perforin pathway are the two main mechanisms by which cytotoxic T lymphocytes induce cell death in cells expressing foreign antigens. Thirdly, by the infusion of granzyme B by T cells into the keratinocytes. Granzymes are serine proteases that are released from cytoplasmic granules within cytotoxic T cells (and natural killer cells) and whose usual role is to induce apoptosis within virus-infected cells, thus destroying them. [18] Cytotoxic T-cells release a protein called perforin, which attacks the target cells forming multimeric complex (of granzyme B, perforin, and granulysin) that enters cells through the mannose 6-phosphate receptor. [19] Granzyme B is then released, to cause apoptosis by various pathways, including the cleaving of caspases (especially caspase-3), which in turn activates caspase-activated DNase and this enzyme degrades DNA, so inducing the apoptotic cascade culminating in cell death. [18, 19]

4. Development of autoantibodies against self-antigens and the promotion of autoimmunity

The autoimmune nature of OLP is evidenced by the chronic and protracted course of the disease, its later age of onset, its higher prevalence in women, its association with other autoimmune diseases, proven demonstration of the T-cell auto-reactivity and increased auto-cytoxicity against basal keratinocytes, its clinical, histological and immunological similarity to graft-versus host disease (GVHD) and the effectiveness of immunosuppressive therapies. Two theories have been advanced to explain the autoimmune nature of OLP, specifically the loss of self-tolerance of the basal keratinocytes: (1) impaired immune-suppression in OLP due to lack of Transforming Growth Factor-β1 (TGF-β1); and (2) loss of "immune-privilege" in OLP. [14, 20]

Impaired Immune-Suppression in OLP (deficient TGF-β1): TGF-β is believed to be important regulator of the immune system by inducing and increasing the differentiation of both Foxp3+ regulatory T cells (Tregs) (and Th17 cells). FOXP3 (forkhead box P3) also known as scurfin, is a protein involved in immune system responses. A member of the FOX protein family, FOXP3 appears to function as a master regulator (transcription factor) in the development and function of regulatory T cells. [21, 22]

TGF-β also appears to block the activation of lymphocytes and monocyte derived phagocytes. TGF-β1 levels and/or activity may be deficient for some of the following reasons: insufficient numbers of TGF-β1-secreting Th3 regulatory T cells; blockage of TGF-β1secretion; secretion of defective, non-functional TGF-β1; defective or inadequate TGF-β1receptor expression; or defective intracellular downstream signalling from the TGF-β1 receptors. Local overproduction of IFN-γ by Th1 $CD4^+$ T cells in OLP lesions would down-regulate the immunosuppressive effect of TGF-β1and so up-regulate keratinocyte MHC class II expression and CD8+ cytotoxic T cell activity explaining the immune responses to antigens including self antigens and the chronicity of OLP.

Loss of "Immune-Privilege" in OLP: The normal oral epithelium, similar to the eye, testes and placenta, may represent an immune-privileged site, by being able to induce apoptosis of infiltrating T-lymphocytes. In these sites, the stromal cells possess Fas Ligand (CD95L) that can trigger the apoptosis of infiltrating inflammatory and immune cells that express Fas (CD95). [20] Keratinocytes themselves can also trigger T-cell apoptosis by the release of the cytokine TNF-α, which on binding the TNF-receptor-1 of T-cells triggers their apoptosis. Loss or impairment of either of these two mechanisms to induce T-cell apoptosis may have a role in the pathogenesis of OLP.

Langerhans cells may also contribute to the loss of self-tolerance. Langerhans cells phagocytose the apoptotic bodies and debris of basal keratinocytes, but in doing so, may process and present to the $CD4^+$ T helper cells a self-antigen derived from the remains of the basal keratinocyte. In turn, this may activate self-reactive $CD4^+$ T cells that differentiate into Th1 or Th2 phenotypes and promote cell- or antibody-mediated autoimmune reactions against basal keratinocytes, including the stimulation of the cytotoxic T cells against the basal keratinocytes. [14]

5. Role of the humoral immune response

The humoral immune response is thought to have some role in the pathogenesis of OLP, even though it is dominated by the T-cell-mediated immune response. Circulating autoantibodies to desmoglein 1 and 3 have been identified, but again the exact role of such autoantibodies remains uncertain. [23 Further evidence of the potential role of humoral immune response in OLP, is a single case report, dating back to 2008, of full resolution of muco-cutaneous lichen planus with oral and oesophageal involvement, following a course of anti-CD20 monoclonal antibody therapy (rituximab) directed against pre-B and mature B lymphocytes, so preventing their evolution to antibody-releasing plasma cells. [24]

6. Non-specific immune mechanisms in OLP pathogenesis

Some of the T-cells in the T-cell dominant lymphocytic infiltrate so pathognomonic for OLP are not specific or targeted. Their presence may be due to pre-existing inflammation that favours the movement of such non-specific T-lymphocytes into the epithelium, which in turn, causes destruction of the keratinocytes. The mechanisms involved include: (1) basement membrane disruption; (2) increased presence of matrix metalloprotienases (MMP); (3) Chemokine (C-C motif) ligand 5 (CCL5) (previously termed RANTES - Regulated on Activation, Normal T cell Expressed and Secreted) activity; and (4) Mast cell activation and degranulation. [14, 15]

Basement Membrane Disruption: Integrity of the epithelial basement membrane is maintained by the keratinocytes, which release collagen IV and laminin V into the basement membrane zone, but the keratinocytes require a basement membrane-derived signal to prevent their apoptosis. Thus, the basement membrane is needed for keratinocyte survival and its integrity is maintained by the keratinocytes. Apoptosis of the keratinocytes by the CD8+ cytotoxic T-cells results in the loss of the maintenance function by performed the keratinocytes, leading to disruption of the basement membrane, thereby allowing the non-specific T-cell to infiltrate the epithelial cell layers. [14, 23] The disruption of the basement membrane also leads to apoptosis of the keratinocytes, due to the loss basement-membrane derived signal to prevent their apoptosis, and so on. This ongoing, self-perpetuating cycle may explain the chronicity of OLP.

Matrix Metalloprotienases (MMPs): MMP-9 concentrations have been found to be increased in culture supernatants taken from patients with OLP compared with normal controls. [25] MMP-9 is one member of a family of some 20 MMPs identified to date, which are all zinc-containing proteinases. [26] MMP-9 (together with MMP-2) are gelatinases that cleave collagen IV. Other MMPs can cleave collagen IV and laminin. The MMPs are inhibited by tissue inhibitors of metalloproteinases (TIMPs) that form stable complexes with MMPs or pro (precursor) MMP's. [27] T-cells release activators of MMP-9, resulting in disruption of the basement membrane.

Chemokine (C-C Motif) Ligand 5 (CCL5 (RANTES)): CCL5 is a key chemokine released by various cells including, activated T-lymphocytes, oral keratinocytes and mast cells and has a critical role in the recruitment of various immune and inflammatory cells, including lymphocytes, monocytes, eosinophils, basophils and mast cells. CCR1, CCR3 to CCR5, and CCR9 and CCR10 are key cell surface receptors for CCL5 and have also been identified in lichen planus. [28] CCL5 attracts mast cells which degranulate, releasing TNF-α and chymase, which in turn up regulates OLP lesional T-cell release of CCL5, leading again to the development of a self-perpetuating cycle, that further contributes to the chronicity of OLP.

Mast Cell Activation and Degranulation: Mast cells are not only increased in numbers, but most are degranulated in OLP (compared with normal tissues). [14, 23, 28] Mast cell degranulation results in the release of variety of pre-inflammatory mediators, including TNF-α, chymase and typtase. TNF-α can up-regulate endothelial cell adhesion molecules required for the lymphocytes to adhere to luminal surfaces of blood vessels and their subsequent extravasation. Chymase, a mast cell protease, activates MMP-9, so contributing to basement membrane disruption. Both chymase and TNF-α can stimulate CCL5 secretion by lesional T-lymphocytes, which in turn can trigger further mast cell degranulation. [28]

7. Genetic factors

Genetic factors clearly must have a role in the pathogenesis of OLP. Recently, the identification of genetic polymorphisms of cytokine/receptor gene loci has been shown to act as clear-cut genetic risk factors for a number of autoimmune diseases. [29] Polymorphism of several cytokines has been shown to be associated with the clinical presentation of LP. [30] Genetic polymorphisms of the first intron of the promoter gene of interferon-γ and development of oral lesions of LP and an association between the –308A TNF-α allele and the development of cutaneous lesions of LP. [30] The occurrence of OLP has also been linked to MHC class II allele

DR6. in those patients who also have HCV. [31] To date no specific HLA antigen profile has been found associated with idiopathic OLP.

In summary, despite the oral mucosa only being capable of a limited immunological response, the immuno-pathogenesis of OLP is complex. OLP appears to be predominantly a delayed-type IV hypersensitivity reaction, due in large measure to cytotoxic CD8+ T-lymphocyte induced apoptosis of the basal keratinocytes of the oral epithelium. There are also a number of aspects, best characterised as immune-deregulation that leads to a self -inducing, self-perpetuating cycle that may explain the chronicity of OLP. However, despite a limited comprehension of the pathogenesis of OLP, therapeutic stratagems are being pursued, based on this understanding, including the trialling of TNF-α inhibitors, interleukin-1 inhibitors, mast cells stabiliser agents, to prevent their degranulation, and the use of agents that can induce the up-regulation of key immune-suppressive cytokines such as TGF-β and interleukin-8, or the *in-vitro* production of these cytokines for use as therapeutic agents.

8. Clinical manifestations of OLP

The diagnosis of OLP is usually made on clinical features alone. However, careful attention to the clinical history is essential, to ensure assessment, and if warranted, the appropriate management, of the extra-oral manifestations of lichen planus. [1, 32, 33]

OLP is classified morphological into seven different clinical presentations: Predominantly white, usually slightly raised lesions consisting of a (1) reticular form (2) papular, and (3) plaque-form seen in about 23% of patients, [34, 35] the predominantly erythematous presentations, with (4) atrophic mucosa, which is seen in some 40% of patients, (5) ulcerative (erosive) lichen planus, seen in some 37% of presenting patients and the rare (6) vesiculo-bullous form (Figures 2a – 4b). [2] In some 10% of patients have their OLP confined to the gingivae, termed (7) "desquamative gingivitis". This term is a clinical descriptor, used to describe inflammation, with a mix of erythema, erosion and/or ulceration of the gingival tissues and the immediately adjacent alveolar mucosa, not incited by the presence of dental bacterial plaque (Figures 5a and 5b). These latter predominantly erythematous forms of OLP can be associated with significant discomfort requiring either topical and/or systemic immunosuppressive therapy. [33] When patients do present with pain, it usually is not spontaneous, but they tend to complain of mild, but noticeable intolerance to particularly salty, spicy or acidic foods (such as any form of curry) brushing of their teeth, which can be made worse and is generalised, on the use of flavoured toothpastes. Rarely, patients will present with widespread oral mucosal ulceration that is spontaneously very painful and so elicit their presentation. The asymptomatic, predominantly white appearing, striated, papular and plaque forms of OLP tend to be found incidentally during the course of an oral examination. They commonly take the form of minute white papules that gradually enlarge and coalesce to form either a reticular, annular, or plaque-like pattern. A characteristic feature is the presence of slender white lines (Wickham's striae) radiating from the papules. In the reticular form, there is a lace-like network of slightly raised white lines, often interspersed with papules or rings. The plaque-like form may be difficult to distinguish from leukoplakia. Oral lesions of lichen planus may also include bullae, but this is rare. These different forms can merge or coexist in the same patient. [1, 34, 35] The commonest sites are inevitably bilateral and include the buccal mucosa (seen in some 90% of patients), gingiva, dorsal tongue, lateral tongue, labial mucosa and the lower lip. Uncommon sites include the palate (Figure 6), upper lip, and floor of the mouth. [34] The gingivae are commonly the site of erythematous/erosive OLP. Involvement of the gingivae is described clinically as desquamative gingivitis, but is not unique to OLP and may feature in the presentation of other oral dermatoses, especially pemphigoid and pemphigus. [34]

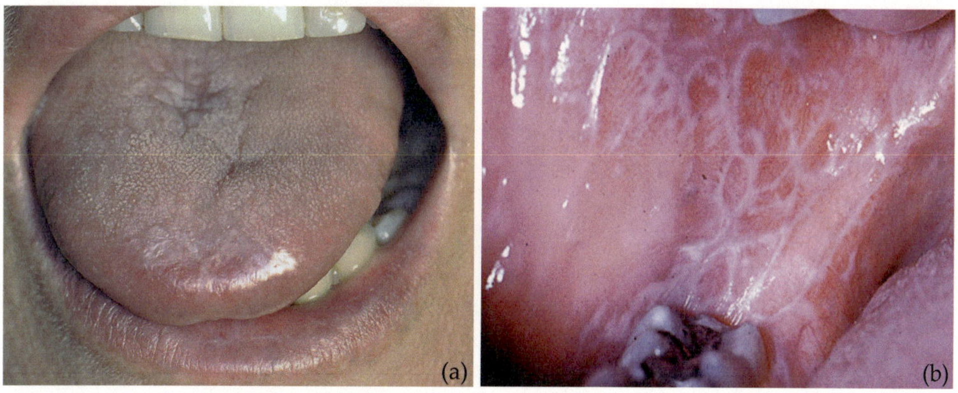

Figure 2. a) Reticular OLP (tongue); b) Reticular OLP (buccal mucosa)

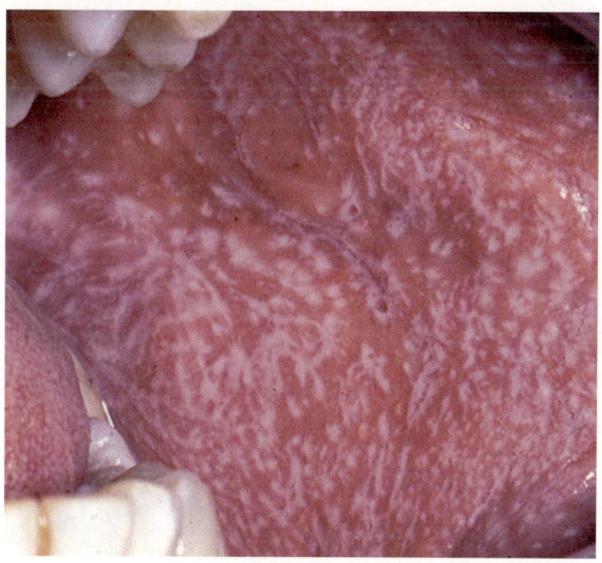

Figure 3. Paupular OLP

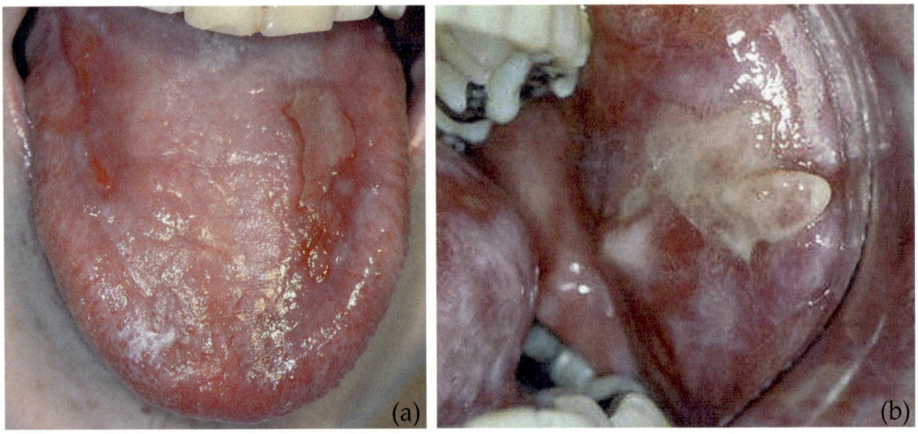

Figure 4. a) Ulcerative (erosive) OLP (dorsal tongue); b) Ulcerative (erosive) OLP (buccal mucosa)

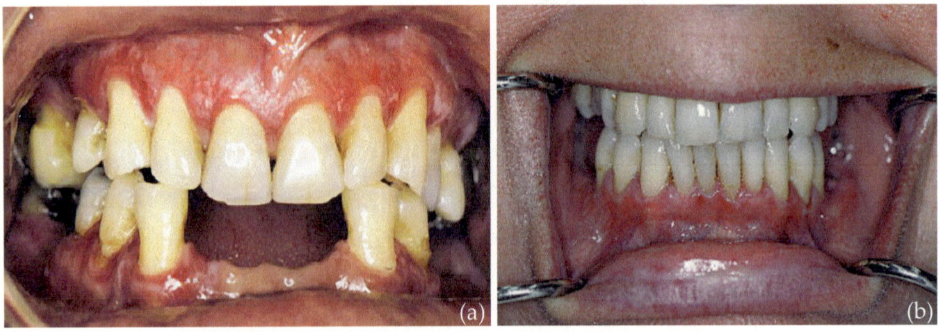

Figure 5. a) Desquamative gingivitis; b) Desquamative gingivitis with plaque form of OLP of central lower lip

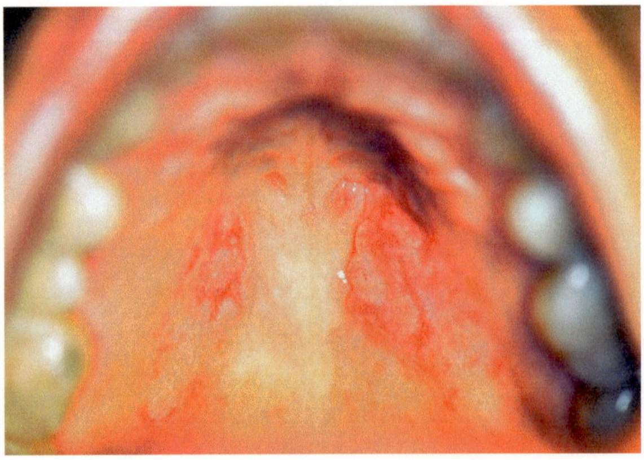

Figure 6. OLP of the hard palate

http://dx.doi.org/10.5772/56482

OLP not only tends to develop in sites of trauma (Koebner phenomenon) but tends to be exacerbated by mechanical factors including biting/chewing habits, dental procedures and rubbing of malpositioned or ill-fitting dentures, teeth and fillings.

9. Clinical subtypes of oral lichenoid reactions

Oral lichenoid reactions encompass several clinical entities. [33-36]

Oral Lichen Planus (OLP): in which patients present with oral lichenoid lesions not readily attributable to any defined cause, that is to say "idiopathic" OLP. OLP represents one aspect of the spectrum of mucocutaneous lichen planus, which can affect potentially any mucosal surface, and/or the skin and its appendages.

Oral Lichenoid Contact Lesions (OLCL): due to allergic contact stomatitis (delayed immune mediated hypersensitivity) and seen in direct topographic relationship to dental restorative materials, most commonly amalgam (Figure 7). [36, 37]

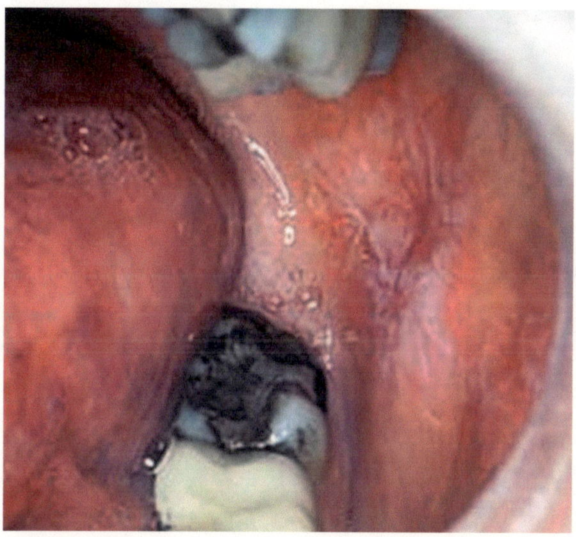

Figure 7. Oral Lichen Contact Lesion (OCLC) – left buccal mucosa

Oral Lichenoid Drug Reactions (OLDR: in which oral and/or cutaneous lesions occur, temporally associated with the taking of certain medications, such as oral hypoglycaemic drugs, angiotensin converting enzyme (ACE) inhibitors, and non-steroidal anti-inflammatory agents (NSAIDS), but historically has been seen with the previous more wide-spread use of gold salts and penicillamine for the management of rheumatoid arthritis. [38]

Oral Lichenoid Lesions of Graft versus Host Disease (OLL-GVHD): in the setting of patients with acute, but predominantly, chronic graft versus host disease (cGVHD). [33]

Lichenoid responses or reactions ("lichenoid stomatitis") of the oral cavity may also be noted with other autoimmune or inflammatory diseases including connective tissue diseases and other immuno-bullous disorders. The cause(s) of the various oral lichenoid lesions, ranging from idiopathic oral lichen planus (OLP) to the "contact" lesion, is not understood, but all the lesions are characterized histologically by a typical "lichenoid tissue reaction" culminating in a common pathologic process, that of T-lymphocyte directed, immune mediated, damage to the oral epithelial basal cells. [1,2]

The diagnosis of OLP is usually made on clinical features alone. However, careful attention to the clinical history is essential, to ensure assessment, and if warranted, the appropriate management, of the extra-oral manifestations of lichen planus (Figures 8a and 8b). [1, 33-35]

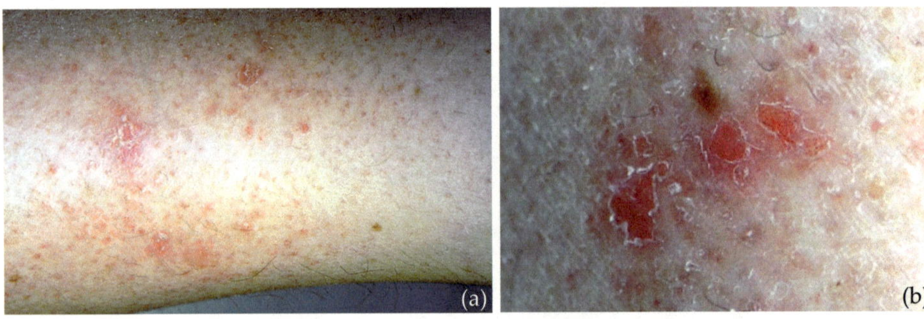

Figure 8. a) LP of the skin; b) LP of the skin (close up)

10. Special investigations

Biopsy (Histopathological and Direct Immune-Fluorescence Investigations (DIF)): The clinical features alone may be sufficiently diagnostic, particularly when presenting with the "classic" reticular form. The evidence regarding the need and value of biopsy for histological confirmation of the diagnosis is not definitive. Studies have shown variability in both inter-observer and intra-observer reliability in the clinicopathological assessment of OLP. [39] As OLP is a chronic disorder that often requires long-term treatment and monitoring, biopsy would be prudent clinical practice, particularly when the disease does not present with its typical manifestations, or when there is concern and therefore need, to exclude dysplasia or malignancy. [1] Furthermore, in severe disease warranting treatment with high-dose systemic corticosteroid therapy or potent "'steroid-sparing" immune-suppressant agents, then a confirmatory biopsy would be appropriate. The histopathological features are shown in Table 1. The findings on direct immune-fluorescence (DIF) are of a fibrin deposition in a linear pattern in the basement membrane zone. Colloid bodies may be positive for fibrin, IgM, and C3. The DIF findings, however, are not diagnostic of OLP, but DIF is certainly useful in differentiating OLP from other oral dermatoses, such as pemphigoid, or immune disorders, such as lupus (both discoid and systemic lupus) given their similar clinical presentation in the oral cavity. [34]

Essential Features (for histopathological diagnosis):

• Signs of "liquefaction degeneration" in the basal cell layer

• Presence of well-defined bandlike zone of cellular infiltration confined to the superficial part of the connective tissue, consisting mainly of T-lymphocytes

• Normal epithelial maturation pattern (absence of epithelial dysplasia)

Non-Essential Histopathological Features that may also be seen:

"Candle-dripping" or "saw-tooth"-like rete ridge conformation

Parakeratosis

Civatte bodies

Separation of epithelium from lamina propria due to basal cell destruction

Exclusionary Histopathological Features (the presence of which would preclude a definitive histopathological diagnosis of OLP).

•Epithelial Dysplasia/Atypia

→Atypical cytomorphology

→Nuclear enlargement or hyperchromasia

→Prevalent dyskeratosis

→Increased number of mitotic figures; aberrant mitosis

→Disordered stratification

•Heterogeneous inflammatory infiltrate

Heterogeneous inflammatory infiltrate with plasma cells and eosinophils

Deep extension below superficial stroma

or perivascular infiltration

• Blunt rete ridges

Table 1. Histopathological features of OLP (adapted from Eisenberg, E. Clinicopathologic patterns of oral lichenoid lesions. Oral Maxillofac Surg Clin North Am, 1994, 6, 445.) [3] (Figures 9a, 9b and 9c)

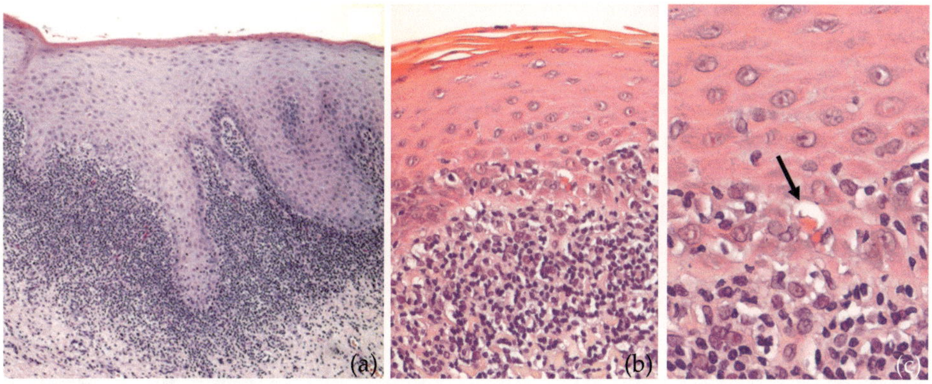

Figure 9. a) Histopathology (low power) band-like inflammatory infiltrate; b) Histopathology – vacuolar degeneration of the basal keratinocytes; c) Histopathology – civatte body

Laboratory Investigations: Generally are not required, except in patients with severe OLP warranting high-dose systemic corticosteroids, with the need to exclude underlying latent infectious diseases that can be reactivated by the corticosteroids (HIV, Hepatitis B and C, and tuberculosis). Again generally not required, except if considering treatment with a suitable 'steroid-sparing systemic agent (e.g.: hydroxychloroquine (Plaquenil), azathioprine or methotrexate) then routine full blood count, and assessment of liver and renal function may be warranted, for baseline assessment and monitoring in patients needing long-term management. [33]

Patch Testing and the Removal of Lichenoid-Inducing Dental Restorative Materials: Idiopathic OLP needs to be distinguished from oral lichenoid contact lesions (OLCL), most commonly seen in direct topographic relationship with amalgam. Cutaneous patch testing, undertaken by a clinician skilled and experienced in "reading" the cutaneous response to a variety of test agents can be useful to confirm the diagnosis of a OLCL, [36, 37] especially in severe, symptomatic cases, in which wide-spread replacement of the amalgam fillings is being considered, given the expense in time and money to the patient concerned. The benefit of such patch testing is to ensure that the alternate dental restorative materials also, in turn, do not incite a lichenoid contact reaction (e.g.: as has been seen with gold and even composite materials). In select cases, and if practical, consideration should be given to the replacement of those isolated restorations, seemingly to be in direct topographic relationship with a lichenoid oral mucosal lesion, particularly if symptomatic, with an alternate material, but the patient needs to be counselled that this may not necessarily prove beneficial. As an interim step, temporary coverage of the suspecting inciting material may be considered to determine if resolution of the OLCL occurs before undertaking definitive removal and replacement of the suspected inciting material.

Additional Measures: Referral for examination by a dermatologist or gynaecologist should be considered, depending on the presenting signs and symptoms reported by the patient.

11. Differential diagnoses

There is a spectrum of oral lesions that resembles OLP both clinically and histopathologically. [33, 34] These "lichen planus–like" ("lichenoid") lesions include the following conditions: (1) Oral lichenoid contact lesions (OLCL) as a result of allergic contact stomatitis (delayed immune mediated hypersensitivity). They are seen in direct topographic relationship to dental restorative materials, such as amalgam. In regards to the approach to oral lichenoid contact lesions, the value of patch testing remains controversial. (2) Oral lichenoid drug reactions (OLDR), wherein oral and/or cutaneous lesions arise in temporal association with the taking of certain medications, for example, oral hypoglycaemic agents, angiotensin-converting enzyme inhibitors, and non-steroidal anti-inflammatory agents. Confirmation of the diagnosis of an oral lichenoid drug reaction may be difficult, since empiric withdrawal of the suspected drug and/or its substitution by an alternative agent may be complicated. [38] (3) Oral lichenoid lesions (OLL-GVHD) of graft-versus-host disease are confined to allogeneic haematopoietic stem transplant recipients who have developed acute, or more commonly, chronic graft-versus-host disease (cGVHD). There is evidence that there is a greater risk of malignant transformation with OLL-GVHD than seen with OLP. [40]

The oral presentation of discoid lupus erythematosus (DLE) can also present with reticular or plaque-like lesions, but it is an uncommon condition that tends to present very much unilaterally, so meriting biopsy for histopathological and direct immune-fluorescence investigations, the latter being most useful in distinguishing OLP from DLE. [34]

11.1. Treatment

An essential first step is patient education as to the chronic nature of OLP and that therapy is not curative, but directed at relieving their symptoms. For treatment to be effective, patients need educated regarding the need to be patient and persistent with the recommended therapy. Instilling in patients the need for ongoing monitoring, not only for patients' response to treatment, but for malignant transformation is also important.

11.2. Supportive measures

The elimination of precipitating or provoking factors is an important initial step in the management of symptomatic OLP. The undertaking of active measures to resolve or minimize mechanical trauma from dental procedures, sharp cusps, rough dental restorations, and ill-fitting prostheses, or chemical trauma from acidic, spicy, or strongly flavoured foods and beverages should be encouraged. Of themselves, such supportive measures can lead to symptomatic improvement, or, more rarely, resolution of the disease.

The accumulation of bacterial plaque, often as a result of the discomfort associated with oral hygiene procedures in patients with gingival involvement, may also exacerbate the condition. The use of supplemental oral hygiene measures, including the use of alcohol-free chlorhexidine gluconate mouth rinses, may be helpful in such cases. [41]

11.3. Pharmacotherapy

Given the immune-mediated aetiology of OLP (and similar conditions such as mucous membrane pemphigoid (MMP)), the aim of therapy, is to minimise or "restrain" the body's immune-mediated inflammatory response, but without risking the activation of opportunistic infections. Treatment should be kept as simple as possible and should not inordinately burden the patient with expensive, complex, unwieldy or protracted treatments that result in non-compliance; therefore, topical corticosteroids remain the mainstay of treatment. [1, 33] Unfortunately, there are only limited evidence-based studies regarding the therapeutic interventions in OLP, and so treatment remains largely empirical. [1]

Topical Treatment:Home Remedies and Over-the-Counter (OTC) Preparations: patient prepared "salty" (saline) mouthwashes are of very limited clinical utility, somewhat palliative, and do not address the aetiological factors seen in OLP, but may facilitate oral hygiene. Patients also often self-prescribe and use any of the variety of OTC anti-microbial mouthwashes, in the mistaken understanding that OLP may be infective in nature, but often complain of their astringency, especially the alcohol containing mouthwashes (and a useful clue as to the diagnosis).

Kenalog in Orabase® is one topical corticosteroid (0.1% triamcinolone) preparation that has the distinct advantage of being mixed with a vehicle for applying medication to the oral surfaces – Orabase® (composed of gelatin, pectin and carmellose in a Plastibase (hydrocarbon gel ointment base)). [1] The use of such an adhesive addresses an important therapeutic issue in treating OLP; that is having sufficient "contact time" between the medicament and the mucosal lesion(s) of OLP. It maintains the medication in close contact with the lesion and provides a protective covering that augments the effects of the corticosteroid. [33]

Prescription Treatments: Topical Corticosteroid Preparations. Topical corticosteroids come in a range of strengths, rated from mild – e.g.: hydrocortisone, to moderate – e.g.: betamethasone valerate, to highly potent, e.g.; clobetasone and means of delivery: pastes, ointments, gels or as inhaled agents (as used in asthma treatment). All agents, used in a variety of delivery methods have demonstrated some efficacy in treating OLP.[1] However, the basic principles guiding topical corticosteroids therapy, is firstly, to use the lowest strength agent possible to achieve a therapeutic benefit, and secondly, for oral mucosal lesions, (as opposed to skin conditions) to favour the use of adhesive containing preparations to prolong contact time, and so avoid the agent being simply washed away by the ever-present saliva.

Compounded Preparations: Empirically, patients report modest to good responses, to the use of moderate, to highly potent topical corticosteroids such as betamethasone valerate mixed with an equal amount (by weight) of Orobase, used 3-4 times daily (after meals) given they are suitably adhesive. One limitation is that they often need to be prepared by specialist compounding pharmacists. A second limitation is that many patients often complain how unpleasant and "tacky" they find this mixture. Use of specially fabricated modified topical fluoride trays, with extended coverage of the gingiva and adjacent alveolar mucosa to hold topical agents in place in the treatment of the desquamative gingivitis form of OLP are reported to be helpful, but again, patient compliance can be poor. [1]

Potent corticosteroids, such as dexamethasone, compounded as a mouthwash suspension (0.1% strength - 40 mg Dexamethasone mixed with 400 ml sterile water) are better tolerated by patients. However, patients must be carefully instructed in their use, emphasising that it is to be used as rinse, for at least 3 minutes (for sufficient therapeutic contact time), at most four times a day (after meals) and to spit out well, to minimise systemic uptake of this highly potent corticosteroid and thereby avoid its adverse effects.

Antifungal Agents: supplemental use of an antifungal agents, such as Daktarin® (miconazole) Oral Gel, or chlorhexidine-containing mouthwashes is warranted given the risk of candidial overgrowth and possible infection secondary to the use of the corticosteroids (whether they be used topically or systemically).

Systemic Agents: Corticosteroids: systemic corticosteroids are used in two ways mainly: firstly, as short-term "pulse" dose of prednisolone up to 0.5 mg per kilogram (of the patient's) body weight for a short period of time (i.e.: 4 days or less and then rapidly tapered) to bring about control of severe ulcerative OLP or in patients with multiple, highly active, sites of lichen planus. Secondly, longer-term, to supplement topical therapies, at sub-physiological doses (equal or less than 7.5 mg prednisone (or equivalent) daily). [1] Monitoring for the principle side-effects (and other adverse effects) of systemic corticosteroid therapy, such as, hypertension, cataract formation, diabetes mellitus, gastric ulceration, osteoporosis, and infection, is needed.

Corticosteroid Alternatives: Retinoids (Topical and Systemic): overall, the published studies suggest that retinoids are potentially effective in the treatment of OLP, but probably inferior to corticosteroids. [42] Systemic retinoids are associated with a number of serious adverse effects that would prohibit their routine use for the management of OLP, and include elevated/deranged transaminase levels, hyper-lipidemia, cheilitis, dryness and desquamation of the skin, alopecia, and dystrophic nail formation, and as well, being teratogenic and therefore their use in women of childbearing age would be contraindicated.

Topical Calcineurin Inhibitors. Cyclosporine, is one of the oldest such agents, but it is relatively expensive and unpleasant tasting, with studies showing an improvement in the oral symptoms that is not significantly better than 1% triamcinolone paste. [43]

Tacrolimus and pimecrolimus are newer calcineurin inhibitors, [44] with an improved safety profile in comparison with cyclosporine, but there are only limited studies as to their benefits, they are expensive and the United States Food and Drug Administration (FDA) has a "Black Box" warning attached to the use of these agents because of a theoretical increased risk of malignancy (squamous cell carcinoma and lymphoma) in patients using topical tacrolimus/pimecrolimus for cutaneous psoriasis. Therefore, the use of these agents should be restricted and patients should be made aware of these concerns. [45]

Phototherapy: there is one study of the benefits of phototherapy using psoralen ultraviolet A light (PUVA) and was included in a recent Cochrane review. However, UV light has a known oncogenic potential and therefore, its use for OLP is questionable. [46

Other and/or "Steroid-Sparing" Systemic Medications: These agents are indicated in patients with refractory LP, confined to the oral cavity, or also involving extra-oral sites, requiring systemic corticosteroids for control. There is only limited evidence supportive of only few potentially useful agents and the use of such agents is best restricted to clinicians highly familiar with these drugs and importantly their adverse effects: (1) *Lysosomotropic amines (the antimalarials chloroquine and hydroxychloroquine):* hydroxychloroquine, at doses of 200 to 400 mg daily, has also been shown to be effective for OLP. [47] (2) *Azathioprine* has been reportedly successful as a "steroid-sparing agent" for cutaneous lichen planus, and there is limited published evidence suggesting it may have a similar role in recalcitrant OLP at doses ranging from 1-2 mg per kilogram (patients' bodyweight), daily. [48] (3) *Mycophenolate mofetil (MMF)* has been employed for treatment of OLP. It is a newer immunosuppressive agent introduced for treatment of immune-mediated skin disorders and also for chronic GVHD. [49, 50] Side effects related to its use are consistent seen with other steroid-sparing alternate immune-suppressive therapies, including a risk of infections and malignancy, in particular, lympho-proliferative neoplasms. MMF, at moderate dosage, appears to be more effective than azathioprine in treatment of cutaneous LP. [51] This is probably due to the fact that MMF has also anti-inflammatory properties exerted by inhibition of leukocyte recruitment and adhesion to endothelial cells. MMF has been used for treatment of severe, erosive-ulcerative oral and genital lichen planus recalcitrant to other systemic therapies. [52, 53] It induced complete, long-lasting remissions without flare-ups over a follow-up period of 4 years. However, the improvement of lesions was delayed, evident only after 4–6 week of treatment. No short-or long-term side effects were experienced, except minor gastrointestinal disturbances. (4) *Methotrexate*. Lundqvist et al carried out an open trial with methotrexate, which has an anti-inflammatory and immunomodulating activity, supplemented with steroid ointments for severe erosive lichen. [54] Four patients were given methotrexate in a dosage of 10–15 mg/ week for about 17 months and they all improved their symptoms. This and another case series demonstrated that methotrexate was a well-tolerated and effective treatment for severe OLP. [54, 55] However, there was a delay in the effect of the methotrexate, so ongoing treatment with systemic corticosteroids may be needed, which are then weaned as the methotrexate becomes increasingly effective. (5) *Other Systemic Agents*: a variety of other immune-suppressant or immune-modifying agents have been trialled in OLP, including Dapsone (diamino-diphenyl sulfone – an anti-tuberculotic/anti-leprotic medication), [56] and thalidomide, [57, 58] but only in the context of isolated, case reports.

Evidence for the use of "'steroid-sparing" and/or "alternate" systemic immune-suppressant agents is poor, limited to case series or case reviews and these agents all have significant side effects that would suggest caution in their use for OLP. However, this needs to be balanced against the known and significant adverse side-effects of high dose corticosteroids needed for recalcitrant OLP, or patients with LP active in several sites. The limitation of much of the literature pertaining to the treatment of OLP is the lack of any unified or agreed objective measures for disease activity and outcomes, which needs to be urgently addressed, so that the various treatments used in OLP can be usefully compared.

11.4. Biological therapies

Biologic therapies, more commonly referred to as "biologics", is a medicinal product such as a vaccine, blood or blood component, allergenic, somatic cell, gene therapy, tissue, recombinant therapeutic protein, or living cells that are used as therapeutics to treat diseases. [59] Biologics are produced by means of biological processes involving recombinant DNA technology, rather than being chemically synthesized. These medications are usually one of three types: (1) Substances that are (nearly) identical to the body's own key signalling proteins, for example are the blood-production stimulating protein erythropoietin; (2) Monoclonal antibodies. These are similar to the plasma-cell derived antibodies that are produced in response to infection, but they are "custom-designed" (using hybridoma technology or other methods) and can therefore be made specifically to counteract or block any given substance in the body, or to target any specific cell type, for example rituximab that selectively targets $CD20^+$ B-cells; and (3) Fusion proteins (receptor constructs), usually based on a naturally-occurring receptor linked to the immunoglobulin frame wherein, the receptor provides the construct with detailed specificity, and the immunoglobulin-structure imparts stability and other useful features in terms of pharmacology.

The management of various immune-mediated disorders has been changed dramatically by the advent of biologic therapies. Biologics are designed to target every stage, as presently understood, in the pathogenesis of immune-inflammatory diseases, by either modulation of T-cells and T-cell functions, or cytokines. However, the future use of biologics will depend on whether they have the ability to truly treat and modify disease, to prevent disease progression and chronicity, or, merely offer more sophisticated, but more expensive palliation, a particular concern in chronic conditions, such as OLP. The other concern is by interfering in the fundamental processes of the immune system, are patients at risk of previously rare and indeed fatal infectious disease, such as progressive multifocal leukoencephalopathy, and is this warranted for a disease such as OLP, which is associated with distress and discomfort, but not serious morbidity or mortality. To date, there have only been limited case reports and case series using biologics for OLP. As with other, more potent immune-suppressive agents now used for OLP, caution is required and patience needed to await and observe the benefits, safety and long-term adverse effects of biologic therapies used in immune-mediated diseases with greater morbidity and potential mortality, such as rheumatoid arthritis, Behçet's disease and the inflammatory bowel diseases, before their use in patients with OLP.

The rationale for the use of biologics in OLP is based on our present understanding of that activated CD8+ and CD4+ lymphocytes play a pivotal role in the pathogenesis of OLP and cytokines such as TNF-α, IL-2 and IFN-γ are involved in the activation and persistence of OLP.

Efalizumab (Raptiva): a humanized monoclonal antibody that binds the CD11a subunit of Lymphocyte function-associated antigen-1 (LFA-1). LFA-1 is a T-cell surface molecule and Intercellular Adhesion Molecule-1 (ICAM-1) is its partner molecule. The interaction between LFA-1 and ICAM-1 regulates many normal T-cell functions. Binding of efalizumab to CD11a on T cells blocks the interaction between LFA-1 and ICAM-1, thus interfering with T-cell activation, migration and cytotoxic functions. This blockade is reversible, and seemingly does not deplete T cells or cause end-organ toxicity, opportunistic infections or malignancy. [60] Cheng and Mann, in 2006, reported a case of a 54-year-old woman with recalcitrant OLP resistant to topical and systemic corticosteroid therapy treated with efalizumab (Raptiva) reported an improvement of oral and cutaneous lesions at 5 weeks after commencement efalizumab therapy (initial dose of 0.7 mg/kg/week, followed by 1.0 mg/kg per week). [61] However, of interest and concern is that efalizumab has been withdrawn from both the American and European markets over safety concerns following the development of three fatal cases of progressive multifocal leucoencephalopathy (PML), a condition linked to immunosuppression that emerged after 3 years of continuous treatment in patients with psoriasis. [62]

Etanercept (Enbrel): This is an example of a fusion protein, consisting of a fully humanised TNF soluble receptor composed of the extracellular portion of two TNF type II receptors joined to the Fc portion of IgG1. The mechanism of action of etanercept is thought to be its competitive inhibition of TNF binding to cell surface TNF receptor (TNFR), preventing TNF mediated cellular responses by rendering TNF biologically inactive. [63] Etanercept may also modulate biological responses controlled by additional downstream molecules (e.g. cytokines, adhesion molecules or proteinases) that are induced or regulated by TNF. It was the first TNF antagonist approved for treatment of psoriasis and psoriatic arthritis and is administered as subcutaneous injection. Yarom published a case report in 2007 of a 56-year-old woman with resistant to treatment to the usual immune-suppressant drugs and whose diabetes and hypertension precluded the use of high dose corticosteroids. [64] Subcutaneous etanercept (25 mg twice weekly) was administered with a 90% symptomatic improvement lesions documented 4 week after beginning therapy. After 10 weeks, the patients stopped the treatment because of the expense, which highlights another concern with the use of the new biologic therapies, their cost.

Alefacept (Amevive): a recombinant protein that, binds to CD2 on the T cell membrane thereby blocking the costimulatory molecule LFA-3/CD2, inhibiting the activation of $CD4^+$ and $CD8^+$ T cells by interfering and inducing apoptosis of memory-effector T lymphocytes. It is composed of an LFA-3 protein and human IgG1 fragment crystallizable (Fc) domain. [65] The rationale for alefacept use in the treatment of lichen planus is the established role for $CD4^+$ T-cells and alefacept induces T-cells apoptosis through natural-killer cells release of granzyme with a reduction in the $CD4^+$ T-cell lymphocyte numbers. Fivenson et al in 2006, reported two cases of generalized lichen planus, with OLP, treated with alefacept, with both patients having full resolution of their lesions and remaining free of lesions and symptoms with completion of the course alefacept therapy, suggesting that it may have a disease modifying effect, negating the need for ongoing therapy for patients with seemingly recalcitrant lichen planus, including OLP. [66]

Rituximab: was approved for the treatment of malignancy by the US Food and Drug Administration in 1997, has been used in certain B-cell lymphomas and treatment resistant rheumatoid arthritis. It is a chimeric murine–human monoclonal antibody to CD20 that depletes normal as well as malignant B cells. Currently, rituximab has been introduced into therapies of numerous immune-mediated conditions in dermatology. [67] Parmentier et al reported in 2008, successful treatment with rituximab for muco-cutaneous LP with oesophageal involvement. [24] There has been no follow-up cases reported since. It is controversial that rituximab targeting B cells could improve T-cell mediated OLP, but it suggests that the humoral arm of the immune system may have some role in the immune-pathogenesis of OLP.

12. Prognosis and outcome

Protracted involvement is typical for OLP, averaging on 8 years, and ranging up to 20 years. In many cases, OLP inexplicably "burns out" allowing for the cessation of any therapeutic interventions. However, some patients may suffer from the cycle of chronic inflammation followed by healing with scarring, with resultant microstomia, if the bucco-labial mucosa is involved, or loss of buccal sulcal depth, making the provision of oral hygiene by the use of a toothbrush difficult for the patient. In such cases, elective removal of the more posteriorly placed teeth, especially unopposed, non-functional, molar teeth may merit consideration. Plastic surgery interventions to relieve the microstomia are indicated, but are painful and can be of limited benefit (Figure 10).

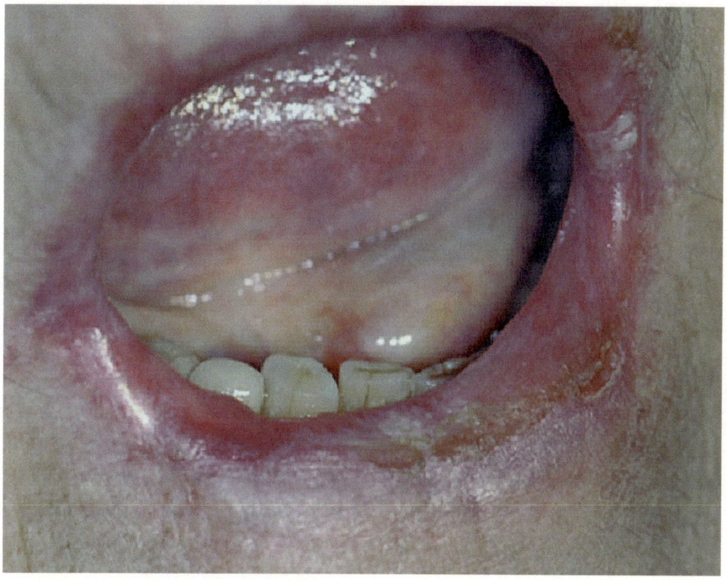

Figure 10. Microstomia secondary to long-standing OLP

12.1. Malignant transformation

The potential for OLP to undergo malignant transformation is controversial. If there is a risk, the risk is very difficult to quantify and possibly so low that it is very difficult to determine if OLP is truly associated with a significant risk for malignant transformation. Prudence would dictate to treat OLP as a potentially malignant lesion. [1, 33] If this approach is favoured, then ongoing, and at the least, annual monitoring, of the oral mucosa, by a clinician experienced in the management of OLP, is indicated. Any lesion suspected to harbour dysplasia and/or frank malignancy (oral squamous cell carcinoma) merits biopsy, and histopathological assessment, preferably by a pathologist experienced in oral pathology. Clinical suspicion should be aroused in the case of a lesion (or lesions) not typical for OLP, a lesion that is heterogeneous in texture and colour (a mixture of erythema and keratosis), or, any isolated area of mucosa that appears to be distinctly unresponsive to therapeutic interventions - such as persistent ulceration - despite clinical improvement in the remainder of the mucosa affected by the OLP. Before undertaking a biopsy, consideration should be given to a trial of topical (and if indicated systemic) corticosteroids and anti-fungal treatments to lessen any associated inflammatory or infectious changes that on histopathological assessment may mask the degree of dysplasia or malignancy within the lesion. [33, 34]

13. Conclusion

Oral lichen planus is a disease that results from CD8+ T cell-mediated apoptosis of basal keratinocytes in response to an unknown endogenous or at times a known exogenous antigen.

The resultant raised white lesions tend to develop in sites of trauma (Koebner phenomenon) and may exhibit the presence of slender white lines (Wickham's striae) radiating from the lesions that are generally asymptomatic, observed often by chance and do not warrant ongoing treatment. However, the predominantly erythematous forms of OLP that is the atrophic, ulcerative (erosive) and desquamative gingivitis presentations of OLP can be significantly symptomatic and warrant treatment. A biopsy is prudent, particularly when the disease does not present with its typical manifestations, or when dysplasia or malignancy needs to be excluded. Signs of "liquefaction degeneration" in the basal cell layer, presence of a well-defined band-like zone of cellular infiltration confined to the superficial part of the connective tissue consisting mainly of T-lymphocytes and normal epithelial maturation pattern are hallmarks of OLP. Patch testing may be employed by a specialist with sufficient expertise in the area to differentiate between idiopathic OLP and oral lichenoid contact lesions OLCL if for instance amalgam is suspected as an allergen.

Therapy, for symptomatic patients, initially should focus on patient education on the elimination of precipitating or provoking factors. Pharmacotherapies are largely empirical and initially potent topical corticosteroids (betamethasone in Orobase, clobetasone in Orobase, or dexamethasone as a mouthwash suspension) are trialled. Topical calcineurin inhibitors are effective but inferior to topical corticosteroids. Low-dose systemic corticosteroids are useful. Hydroxychloroquine, azathioprine, methotrexate, and mycophenolate may be effective in refractory disease. The efficacy (as well as their long-term safety) of biologic agents remains to better evaluated by larger, prospective studies.

OLP inexplicably burns out after a mean period of 8 years. The risk of malignancy is controversial but regular surveillance is advisable with biopsies of suspicious areas recommended to detect early dysplastic changes.

Author details

Mark Schifter[1,2], Suran L. Fernando[3,4] and Jamma Li[4]

1 Department of Oral Medicine, Oral Pathology and Special Care Dentistry, Westmead Hospital, Western Sydney, Australia

2 Faculty of Dentistry, University of Sydney, Sydney, NSW, Australia

3 Department of Clinical Immunology and Allergy, Royal North Shore Hospital, Sydney, Australia

4 Sydney Medical School – Northern, Sydney University, Sydney, Australia

Department of Clinical Immunology and Allergy, Royal North Shore Hospital, Sydney, Australia

References

[1] Al-Hashimi I, Schifter M, Lockhart PB, Wray D, Brennan M, Migliorati CA, et al. Oral lichen planus and oral lichenoid lesions: diagnostic and therapeutic considerations. Oral Surg Oral Med Oral Pathol Oral Radiol Endod 2007;103:S25:1-12.

[2] Andreasen JO. Oral lichen planus. 1. A clinical evaluation of 115 cases. Oral Surg Oral Med Oral Pathol; 1968; 25: 31–42.

[3] Eisenberg, E. Clinicopathologic patterns of oral lichenoid lesions. Oral Maxillofac Surg Clin North Am, 1994, 6, 445.

[4] Staubach P. Lichen planus. CME Dermatol 2009; 4: 68-79.

[5] Wilson, E. On lichen planus. J Cutan Med Dis Skin 1869; 3: 117-132.

[6] Miller RAW. The Koebner phenomenon. Int J Dermatol 1982;21:192-7.

[7] Wickham, LF. Sur un signe pathognomonique delichen du Wilson (lichen plan) stries et punctuations grisatres. Ann Dermatol Syph 1895; 6: 17-20.

[8] Hallopeau H. Sur un cas de lichen de Wilson gingival avec neoplasia voisine dans la région maxillaire. Bull Soc Fr Dermatol Syphiligr 1910;17:32.

[9] Bouquot JE, Gundlach KK. Oral exophytic lesions in 23,616 white Americans over 35 years of age. Oral Surg Oral Med Oral Pathol 1986: 62: 284–291.

[10] McCartan BE, Healy CM. The reported prevalence of oral lichen planus: a review and critique. J Oral Pathol Med 2008; 37:447–53.

[11] Axe'll T, Rundquist L. Oral lichen planus – a demographic study. Community Dent Oral Epidemiol 1987; 15: 52–6.

[12] Sugerman PB, Savage NW, Walsh LJ, et al. The pathogenesis of oral lichen planus. Crit Rev Oral Biol Med. 2002; 13: 350-65.

[13] Lodi G, Scully C, Carrozzo M, Griffiths M, Sugerman PB, Thongprasom K. Current controversies in oral lichen planus; report of an international consensus meeting-Part 1. Viral infections and aetiopathopathogenesis. Oral Surg Oral Med Oral Pathol Oral Radiol Endod 2005;100:40-51.

[14] Sugerman PB, Satterwhite K, Bigby M. Autocytotoxic T-cell clones in lichen planus. Br J Dermatol 2000;142:449-56.

[15] http://www.dako.com/au/ar38/p104620/prod_products.htm

[16] Khan A, Farah CS, Savage NW, et al. Th1 cytokines in oral lichen planus. J Oral Pathol Med 2003;32:77-83.

[17] Wajant H. The Fas signaling pathway: more than a paradigm. Science 2002; 296 (5573): 1635–6

[18] Bots M, Medema JP. Granzymes at a glance. J Cell Sci; 2006; 119: 5011–4.

[19] Buzza MS, Bird PI. Extracellular granzymes: current perspectives. Biol Chem 2006; 387: 827–37.

[20] Roopashree MR, Gondhalekar RV, Shashikanth MC, George J, Thippeswamy SH, Shukla A. Pathogenesis of oral lichen planus--a review. J Oral Pathol Med. 2010; 39: 729-34.

[21] Zhang L, Zhao Y. The regulation of Foxp3 expression in regulatory CD4(+)CD25(+)T cells: multiple pathways on the road. J. Cell. Physiol 2007; 211: 590–597

[22] Prime SS, Pring M, Davies M, Paterson IC. TGF-beta signal transduction in oro-facial health and non-malignant disease (part I). Crit Rev Oral Biol Med; 2004; 15: 324-36

[23] Lukacˇ J, Brozovic´ S, Vucˇ ic´evic´-Boras V, et al. Serum autoantibodies to desmogleins 1 and 3 in patients with oral lichen planus. Croat Med J 2006; 47: 53–8.

[24] Parmentier L, Bron BA, Prins C, Samson J, Masouye´ I, Borradori L. Mucocutaneous lichen planus with esophageal involvement: successful treatment with an anti-CD20monoclonal antibody. Arch Dermatol 2008; 144: 1427–30.

[25] Zhou XJ, Sugerman PB, Savage NW, Walsh LJ. Matrix metalloproteinases and their inhibitors in oral lichen planus. J Cutan Pathol 2001; 28: 72–82

[26] Nagase H, Woessner JF. Matrix metalloproteinases. J Biol Chem 1999; 274: 21491–4

[27] Brew K, Dinakarpandian D, Nagase H. Tissue inhibitors of metalloproteinases: evolution, structure and function. Biochim Biophys Acta 2000; 1477: 267–8

[28] Zhao ZZ, Sugerman PB, Zhou XJ, Walsh LJ, Savage NW. Mast cell degranulation and the role of T cell RANTES in oral lichen planus. Oral Dis 2001; 7: 246–51.

[29] Farhi D, Dupin N. Pathophysiology, etiologic factors, and clinical management of oral lichen planus, part I: facts and controversies. Clin Dermatol; 2010: 28:100–108

[30] Carrozzo M, Uboldi de Capei M, Dametto E, et al. Tumor necrosis factor-alpha and interferon-gamma polymorphisms contribute to susceptibility to oral lichen planus. J Invest Dermatol 2004;122: 87-94.

[31] Carrozzo M, Francia Di Celle P, Gandolfo S, et al. Increased frequency of HLA-DR6 allele in Italian patients with hepatitis C virus-associated oral lichen planus. Br J Dermatol 2001; 144: 803-8.

[32] Schlosser BJ. Lichen planus and lichenoid reactions of the oral mucosa. Dermatol Ther 2010; 23: 251–267.

[33] Schifter M, Yeoh SC, Coleman H, Georgiou A. Oral mucosal diseases: the inflammatory dermatoses. Aust Dent J: 2010: 55 Suppl 1: 23-38.

[34] Eisen D. The clinical features, malignant potential, and systemic associations of oral lichen planus: a study of 723 patients. J Am Acad Dermatol 2002: 46: 207–214.

[35] Sugerman PB, Savage NW, Zhou X, Walsh LJ, Bigby M. Oral lichen planus. Clin Dermatol 2000;18:533-539.

[36] Lopez-Jornet P, Camacho-Alonso F, Gomez-Garcia F, Bermejo Fenoll A. The clinicopathological characteristics of oral lichen planus and its relationship with dental materials. Cont Dermatol 2004;51:210-211.

[37] Thornhill MH, Pemberton MN, Simmons RK, Theaker ED. Amalgam-contact hypersensitivity lesions and oral lichen planus. Oral Surg Oral Med Oral Pathol Oral Radiol Endod 2003;95:291-299.

[38] McCartan BE, McCreary CE. Oral lichenoid drug eruptions. Oral Dis 1997;3:58-63.

[39] Van der Meij EH, Van der Waal I. Lack of clinicopathologic correlation in the diagnosis of oral lichen planus based on the presently available diagnostic criteria and suggestions for modification. J Oral Pathol Med 2003;32:507-512.

[40] Curtis RE, Metayer C, Rizzo JD, Socie G, Sobocinski KA, Flowers ME, et al. Impact of chronic GVHD therapy on the development of squamous-cell cancers after hematopoietic stem-cell transplantation: an international case-control study. Blood 2005;105:3802-3811.

[41] Holmstrup P, Schiotz AW, Westergaard J. Effect of dental plaque control on gingival lichen planus. Oral Surg Oral Med Oral Pathol 1990;69:585-590.

[42] Giustina TA, Stewart JC, Ellis CN, Regezi JA, Annesley T, Woo TY, et al. Topical application of isotretinoin gel improves oral lichen planus. Arch Dermatol 1986;122:534-536.

[43] Sieg P, Von Domarus H, Von Zitzewitz V, Iven H, Farber L. Topical cyclosporin in oral lichen planus: a controlled, randomized, prospective trial. Br J Dermatol 1995;132:790-794.

[44] Swift JC, Rees TD, Plemons JM, Hallmon WW, Wright JC. The effectiveness of 1% pimecrolimus cream in the treatment of oral erosive lichen planus. J Periodontol 2005;76:627-635.

[45] Becker JC, Houben R, Vetter CS, Bröcker E. The carcinogenic potential of tacrolimus ointment beyond immune suppression: a hypothesis creating case report. BMC Cancer 2006;6:7-13.

[46] Lundquist G, Forsgren H, Gajecki M, Emtestam L. Photochemotherapy of oral lichen planus. Oral Surg Oral Med Oral Pathol Oral Radiol Endod 1995;79:554-558.

[47] Eisen D. Hydroxychloroquine sulfate (Plaquenil) improves oral lichen planus: an open trial. J Am Acad Dermatol 1993;28:609-612.

[48] Schram ME, Borgonjen RJ, Bik CM, van der Schroeff JG, van Everdingen JJ, Spuls PI; Off-Label Working and Project Group of Dutch Society of Dermatology and Venereology. Off-label use of azathioprine in dermatology: a systematic review. Arch Dermatol 2011: 147: 474-88.

[49] Böhm M, Beissert S, Schwarz T, Metze D, Luger T. Bullous pemphigoid treated with mycophenolate mofetil. Lancet 1997; 349: 541.

[50] Bischoff, M, Kirsten D, Sanchez H, Günzelmann S, Fauser AA. Efficacy and safety of mycophenolate mofetil for the treatment of acute and chronic GVHD in bone marrow transplant recipient. Transplant Proc 1998; 30: 4087–4089.

[51] Nousari HC, Goyal S, Anhalt GJ. Successful treatment of resistant hypertrophic and bullous lichen planus with mycophenolate mofetil. Arch Dermatol 1999; 135: 1420–1421.

[52] Basara N, Blau WI, et al. Successful treatment of resistant hypertrophic and bullous lichen planus with mycophenolate mofetil. Arch Dermatol 1999; 135: 1420–1421.

[53] Frieling U, Bonsmann G, Schwarz T, Luger, TA, Beissert S. Treatment of severe lichen planus with mycophenolate mofetil. J Am Acad Dermatol; 2003; 49: 1063–1066.

[54] Lundqvist NE, Wahlin YB, Hofer PA. Methotrexate supplemented with steroid ointments for the treatment of severe erosive lichen ruber. Acta Derm Venereol 2002; 82: 63–64.

[55] Torti DC, Jorizzo JL, McCarty MA. Oral lichen planus: a case series with emphasis on therapy. Arch Dermatol 2007; 143: 511–515.

[56] Beck HI, Brandrup F. Treatment of erosive lichen planus with dapsone. Acta Derm Venereol 1986; 66: 366–367.

[57] Camisa C, Popovsky JL. Effective treatment of oral erosive lichen planus with thalidomide. Arch Dermatol 2000; 136: 1442–1443.

[58] Macario-Barrel A, Balguerie X, Joly P. Treatment of erosive oral lichen planus with thalidomide. Ann Dermatol Venereol 2003; 130: 1109–1112.

[59] Center for Biologics Evaluation and Research (2007-10-29). "What is a biological product?". U.S. Food and Drug Administration

[60] Gottlieb AB, Gordon KB, Hamilton TK. Maintenance of efficacy and safety with continuous efalizumab therapy in patients with moderate to severe chronic plaque psoriasis: final phase IIIb study results. Poster presented at the 63rd Annual Meeting of the American Academy of Dermatology; February 18-22, 2005, New Orleans, La.

[61] Cheng A, Mann C. Oral erosive lichen planus treated with efalizumab. Arch Dermatol 2006 142; 680–682.

[62] Rustin MH. Long-term safety of biologics in the treatment of moderate-to-severe plaque psoriasis: review of current data. Br J Dermatol 2012; 167 Suppl 3: 3-11

[63] Spencer-Green G. Etanercept (Enbrel): update on therapeutic use. Ann Rheum Dis 2000; 59 Suppl 1: 146–149.

[64] Yarom, N. Etanercept for the management of oral lichen planus. Am J Clin Dermatol 2007; 8: 121.

[65] New drugs. Australian Prescriber 2004; 27: 5

[66] Fivenson DP, Mathes B. Treatment of generalized lichen planus with alefacept. Arch. Dermatol 2006; 142: 151–152.

[67] Carr DR, Heffernan MP. Innovative uses of rituximab in dermatology. Dermatol Clin 2010; 28: 547–57.